Nanocellulose Materials

Isamu Ogura • Katsuhide Fujita
Editors

Nanocellulose Materials

Health and Environmental Safety Perspectives

Springer

Editors
Isamu Ogura
Research Institute of Science for Safety and Sustainability
National Institute of Advanced Industrial Science and Technology (AIST)
Tsukuba, Ibaraki, Japan

Katsuhide Fujita
Research Institute of Science for Safety and Sustainability
National Institute of Advanced Industrial Science and Technology (AIST)
Tsukuba, Ibaraki, Japan

ISBN 978-981-92-2147-9 ISBN 978-981-92-2148-6 (eBook)
https://doi.org/10.1007/978-981-92-2148-6

This book is a translation of the original Japanese edition, "Cellulose Nanofiber no Anzensei Hyoukasho 2025 (Safety Assessment Report on Cellulose Nanofibers 2025)", published by the National Institute of Advanced Industrial Science and Technology (AIST). The original publication was publicly released on the website https://www.aist.go.jp/aist_j/news/announce/pr20250127.html in 2025.

This Springer imprint is published by the registered company Springer Nature Singapore Pte Ltd.
The registered company address is: 152 Beach Road, #21-01/04 Gateway East, Singapore 189721, Singapore

Preface

The increasing use of nanocellulose materials (NCMs), including cellulose nanofibrils (CNFs)—also referred to as cellulose nanofibers (CNFs) or nano-fibrillated cellulose (NFC)—and cellulose nanocrystals (CNCs), has attracted significant attention because these materials offer exceptional performance and sustainability. CNFs, for example, are biomass-derived materials that weigh roughly one-fifth as much as steel while exhibiting more than five times its strength. NCMs are expected to accelerate applications across diverse industries, not only as alternatives to petroleum-based materials but also as key contributors to achieving a carbon-neutral society, given their origin from renewable resources such as wood, which absorbs and fixes atmospheric carbon dioxide.

However, industrial nanomaterials possess unique physical characteristics—such as extremely small particle sizes and distinctive morphologies—that raise concerns about potential adverse health effects differing from those of conventional chemical substances. Scientifically assessing and confirming the safety of new materials prior to their implementation in society is indispensable and has become a major international priority. Moreover, even when a material exhibits low toxicity and limited exposure risk, insufficient safety information may lead to public misunderstanding or reputational damage, placing the material at a disadvantage in competitive markets. This issue is particularly relevant for fibrous nanomaterials, for which inadequate safety data may prompt precautionary regulatory actions similar to those applied to asbestos, requiring stringent exposure controls.

NCMs are naturally derived industrial nanomaterials with unique characteristics that distinguish them from previously assessed nanomaterials. CNFs, for instance, exhibit high viscosity and considerable diversity with respect to raw materials, surface modifications, degree of fibrillation, and the type and amount of impurities. Composed of glucose-based linear polymers originating from plants, nanocellulose lacks distinctive elemental signatures and exhibits low absorbance, making separation, identification, detection, and quantification from other components challenging. Owing to these properties, conventional evaluation methods developed for other industrial nanomaterials cannot be directly applied, necessitating the development of new testing methods and measurement techniques.

In response to this need, the National Institute of Advanced Industrial Science and Technology (AIST), in collaboration with Oji Holdings Corporation, DKS Co. Ltd., Daio Paper Corporation, and Nippon Paper Industries Co., Ltd., conducted a Japanese national research project commissioned by the New Energy and Industrial Technology Development Organization (NEDO) titled *Development of Technology for Manufacturing Processes of Chemicals Derived from Inedible Plants/Development of Safety Assessment Methods for CNFs* (JPNP13006) from fiscal years 2017 to 2019. This project focused on three types of CNFs and involved the development of methods for detection and quantification, intratracheal administration, skin permeability testing, and emission and exposure assessments. The results were compiled into publicly available resources, including *Examples of Detection and Quantification of Cellulose Nanofibers* (Japanese version), *A Manual for Toxicity Testing of Cellulose Nanofibers* (Japanese and English versions), and *Examples of Emission and Exposure Assessment of Cellulose Nanofibers and Their Applied Products* (Japanese version) (Fig. 1, https://riss.aist.go.jp/results-and-dissemin/1625/).

Subsequently, a second NEDO project titled *Cellulose Nanofiber-Related Technology Development to Contribute to a Carbon Cycle Society / Development of CNF Utilization Technology/Development of Hazard Assessment Methods and Safety Assessment for Various Product Applications* (JPNP20009) was carried out from fiscal years 2020 to 2024. Within this project, AIST undertook the following activities:

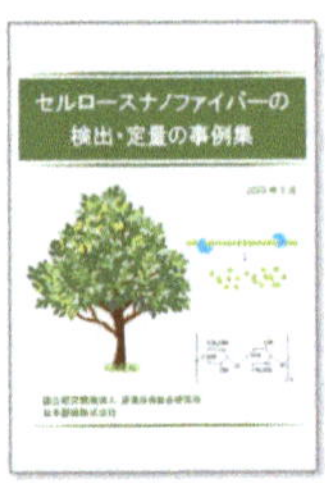

1. Examples of Detection and Quantification of Cellulose Nanofibers (Japanese version)

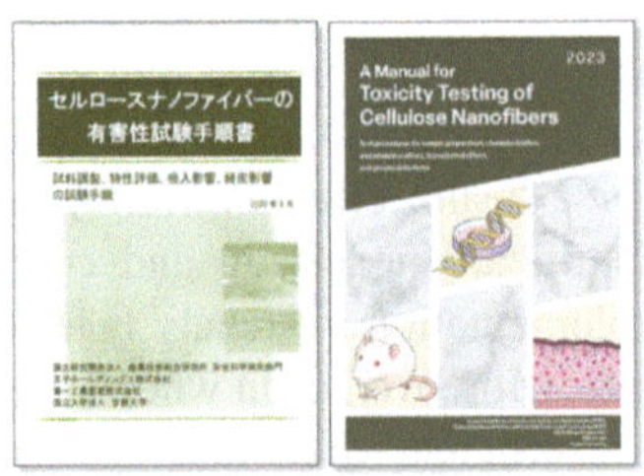

2. A Manual for Toxicity Testing of Cellulose Nanofibers (Japanese and English versions)

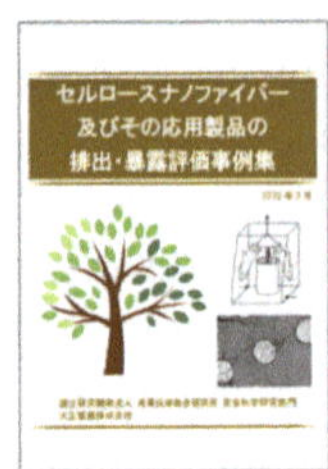

3. Examples of Emission and Exposure Assessment of Cellulose Nanofibers and Their Applied Products (Japanese version)

Fig. 1 Documents related to CNF safety assessment methods and evaluation results1. Examples of Detection and Quantification of Cellulose Nanofibers (Japanese version, published March 2020): An overview of analytical methods for detecting and quantifying CNFs, including acid hydrolysis, enzymatic hydrolysis, and thermal decomposition. The document provides detailed procedures, measurement examples, and key considerations2. A Manual for Toxicity Testing of Cellulose Nanofibers (Japanese and English versions, published 2023): Compilation of procedures for sample preparation, characterization, inhalation testing, and dermal testing for CNF toxicity assessment, along with evaluation results and findings obtained using these methods3. Examples of Emission and Exposure Assessment of Cellulose Nanofibers and Their Applied Products (Japanese version, published March 2020): A summary of emission and exposure assessment results for CNFs and CNF-based products, including on-site investigations, simulated emission tests of CNF powders and composites, and evaluations of CNF biodegradability

1. Inhalation toxicity assessment using cultured cells applicable to a wide range of CNF types
2. Evaluation of potential mesothelioma risk comparable to that associated with asbestos
3. Ecotoxicity evaluation targeting aquatic organisms (e.g., algae, crustaceans, and fish)
4. Emission and exposure assessment of various CNFs and their applied products

Whereas the 2017–2019 project primarily focused on developing methodologies required for the safety evaluation of three representative CNF types, the 2020–2024 project expanded both the range of CNFs examined and the scope of the evaluation, primarily aiming at obtaining specific assessment results. Furthermore, the latter project included participation from the University of Fukui alongside AIST and incorporated *in vivo* studies evaluating biological safety following inhalation and oral exposure.

To support businesses handling CNFs, as well as those developing CNF-based applications, AIST compiled the findings of the NEDO projects on CNF safety assessment together with a comprehensive review of the scientific literature and published the *Safety Assessment Report on Cellulose Nanofibers* (Japanese version) in December 2022, followed by a revised edition in January 2025 (Fig. 2, https://riss.aist.go.jp/results-and-dissemin/1625/). This book is the English translation of that report. Although both the original Japanese report and this book primarily focus on CNFs, they also include broader information on NCMs, including CNCs. It is our hope that this book will contribute to the proper safety management of NCMs and to the development of safe nanocellulose-based products.

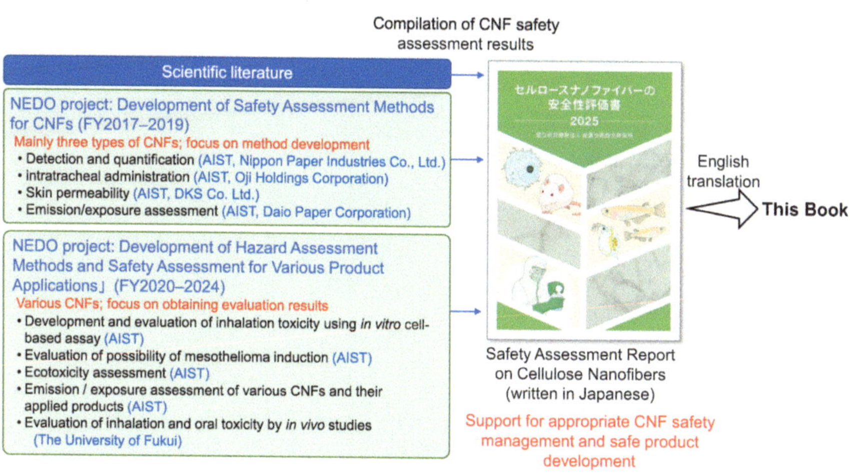

Fig. 2 Summary of information compiled in this book

Important Notice

The research findings presented in this book, obtained through the NEDO projects, do not guarantee the overall safety of NCMs. The International Organization for Standardization (ISO) defines *safety* as a state of freedom from unacceptable risk, where risk is determined by the combination of hazard and exposure. This book organizes information on hazards—such as genotoxicity, mesothelioma, inhalation effects, dermal effects, oral toxicity, and ecological impacts—as well as data on emission and exposure assessment. It should be emphasized that risk cannot be determined solely on the basis of hazard evaluation; comprehensive risk assessment that considers actual exposure conditions is essential.

Furthermore, the evaluation results presented herein are based on specific NCMs and test conditions and should not be interpreted as representative of all NCMs. These findings do not imply that similar results will be obtained under different conditions or applications. Future evaluations should ensure consistency with international assessment frameworks, such as ISO Technical Reports (ISO/TR) and Organisation for Economic Co-operation and Development (OECD) Test Guidelines, to enhance scientific validity and global comparability.

Tsukuba, Ibaraki, Japan

Isamu Ogura
Katsuhide Fujita

The original version of the book has been revised. A correction to this book can be found at https://doi.org/10.1007/978-981-92-2148-6_10

Acknowledgments

This book is based on the research results of the project commissioned by the New Energy and Industrial Technology Development Organization (NEDO): *Cellulose Nanofiber-Related Technology Development to Contribute to a Carbon Cycle Society/Development of CNF Utilization Technology/Development of Hazard Assessment Methods and Safety Assessment for Various Product Applications* (JPNP20009).

Contents

1 **Overview of the Book: Background, Scope, and Key Findings** 1
Isamu Ogura and Katsuhide Fujita

2 **Genotoxicity: Evidence, Mechanisms, and Safety Implications** 9
Katsuhide Fujita

3 **Mesothelioma Potential: Comparative Insights and Safety Findings** 23
Masanori Horie

4 **Inhalation Effects: Pulmonary Responses and Long-Term Considerations** 39
Katsuhide Fujita and Akihiro Moriyama

5 **Dermal Effects: Skin Barrier Interactions and Irritation Potential** 73
Katsuhide Fujita

6 **Oral Toxicity: Experimental Findings and Safety Implications for Nanocellulose** 81
Akihiro Moriyama

7 **Emissions and Exposure: Case Studies and Strategies for Safe Handling of Nanocellulose** 93
Isamu Ogura

8 **Ecotoxicity: Methods, Challenges, and Findings in Assessing Ecological Effects of Nanocellulose** 121
Rie Tai, Isamu Ogura, and Hiroyuki Mano

9 Biodegradability: Effects of Nanosizing and Chemical Modification 151
Isamu Ogura

Correction to: Nanocellulose Materials C1
Isamu Ogura and Katsuhide Fujita

Index 157

Editors and Contributors

About the Editors

Isamu Ogura Research Institute of Science for Safety and Sustainability (RISS), National Institute of Advanced Industrial Science and Technology (AIST), Tsukuba, Ibaraki, Japan

Katsuhide Fujita Research Institute of Science for Safety and Sustainability (RISS), National Institute of Advanced Industrial Science and Technology (AIST), Tsukuba, Ibaraki, Japan

Contributors

Katsuhide Fujita Research Institute of Science for Safety and Sustainability (RISS), National Institute of Advanced Industrial Science and Technology (AIST), Tsukuba, Ibaraki, Japan

Masanori Horie Health and Medical Research Institute, National Institute of Advanced Industrial Science and Technology (AIST), Takamatsu, Kagawa, Japan

Hiroyuki Mano Research Institute of Science for Safety and Sustainability (RISS), National Institute of Advanced Industrial Science and Technology (AIST), Tsukuba, Ibaraki, Japan

Akihiro Moriyama Research Institute of Science for Safety and Sustainability (RISS), National Institute of Advanced Industrial Science and Technology (AIST), Tsukuba, Ibaraki, Japan

Isamu Ogura Research Institute of Science for Safety and Sustainability (RISS), National Institute of Advanced Industrial Science and Technology (AIST), Tsukuba, Ibaraki, Japan

Rie Tai Research Institute of Science for Safety and Sustainability (RISS), National Institute of Advanced Industrial Science and Technology (AIST), Tsukuba, Ibaraki, Japan

Abbreviations

ACC	Aqueous counter collision
AIST	National Institute of Advanced Industrial Science and Technology
Ames test	A bacterial reverse mutation test used to detect chemical-induced point mutations.
Algal growth inhibition test	An ecotoxicity test in which algae (e.g., *Pseudokirchneriella subcapitata*) are exposed to chemicals to assess inhibition of growth rate. OECD TG 201 specifies a 72-h exposure period.
APS	Aerodynamic particle sizer. An instrument that measures aerosol number concentration as a function of aerodynamic diameter, typically in the particle size range of approximately 0.5–20 μm.
Battery test	A genotoxicity assessment strategy combining multiple test methods and/or endpoints.
Cellulose microfibrils (CMFs)	Often used synonymously with cellulose nanofibers (CNFs), depending on the context.
Cellulose nanocrystals (CNCs)	Rod-shaped nanoscale cellulose particles produced by acid hydrolysis of amorphous cellulose regions; also referred to as nanocrystalline cellulose (NCC).
Cellulose nanofibrils or cellulose nanofibers (CNFs)	Cellulose fibers with nanoscale diameters (typically several to ~100 nm), produced by chemical and/or mechanical treatments; also produced by bacteria. Alternative terms include nanofibrillated cellulose (NFC), nanofibrillar cellulose (NFC), microfibrillated cellulose (MFC), microfibrillar cellulose (MFC), and cellulose microfibrils (CMFs).

Chemokine	A subtype of cytokine consisting of small-secreted proteins that induce leukocyte migration and contribute to inflammatory responses.
Chromosomal aberration test	A genotoxicity test detecting structural and numerical chromosomal abnormalities induced by chemicals in cultured mammalian cells.
CNTs	Carbon nanotubes.
Comet assay	A genotoxicity test using single-cell gel electrophoresis to detect DNA strand breaks associated with damage and repair processes.
Comprehensive gene expression analysis	A technique that analyzes changes in the expression of thousands to tens of thousands of genes to assess biological responses to external stimuli.
Condensation particle counter (CPC)	An instrument that measures total aerosol number concentration, typically covering particle sizes from approximately 0.01 μm to >1 μm (with lower size limits down to ~0.001 μm, depending on the model).
Cultured cell test	An *in vitro* test using cells isolated from organisms and cultured in appropriate media for experimental evaluation.
Cytokine	Small secreted proteins that mediate intercellular communication and regulate immune and inflammatory responses.
Daphnia magna reproduction test	A chronic ecotoxicity test in which *Daphnia magna* are exposed to chemicals to evaluate long-term effects based on offspring production. OECD TG 211 specifies a 21-day exposure period.
Daphnia sp. acute immobilisation test	An acute ecotoxicity test in which neonate daphnids are exposed to chemicals, with effects assessed based on immobilization. OECD TG 202 specifies a 48-h exposure period.
DPMFA	Dynamic probabilistic material flow analysis.
EC_{50}	50% effective concentration; the exposure concentration at which 50% of test organisms exhibit a defined effect.

Fish, acute toxicity test	An ecotoxicity test in which juvenile fish (e.g., medaka) are exposed to chemicals to assess short-term effects such as mortality and behavioral abnormalities. OECD TG 203 specifies a 96-h exposure period.
Fish, early-life stage toxicity test	An ecotoxicity test in which fish are exposed from fertilized eggs to early feeding stages to evaluate long-term toxicity. OECD TG 210 specifies an exposure period of approximately 40 days.
Genotoxicity	The ability of a substance to induce structural or quantitative changes in DNA or chromosomes; considered one mechanism underlying carcinogenesis.
Inhalation toxicity test	An *in vivo* test in which laboratory animals (e.g., rats or mice) inhale airborne test substances, followed by evaluation of respiratory and systemic effects.
Intratracheal instillation test	An *in vivo* test in which a suspension of a test substance is directly administered into the trachea of laboratory animals (e.g., rats or mice) using a dosing device to assess pulmonary effects.
In vitro test	Tests conducted using isolated cells, tissues, or biological systems outside a living organism.
In vivo test	Tests conducted in whole living organisms.
ISO	International Organization for Standardization
LC_{50}	50% lethal concentration; the exposure concentration at which 50% of test organisms die.
LD_{50}	50% lethal dose; the administered dose at which 50% of test animals die.
LPS	Lipopolysaccharide; a polysaccharide component of the outer membrane of Gram-negative bacteria; also known as endotoxin.
Macrophage	A type of white blood cell that engulfs and digests bacteria, foreign particles, and cellular debris.
Mesothelial cell	Thin epithelial-like cells that line the pleura, peritoneum, and pericardium.
Mesothelioma	A malignant tumor, typically of the pleura or peritoneum, strongly associated with asbestos exposure.

Microcrystalline cellulose (MCC)	A highly purified, partially depolymerized cellulose produced by acid hydrolysis, typically present as micron-sized particles and widely used in pharmaceuticals and food applications.
Microfibrillated cellulose or microfibrillar cellulose (MFC)	Often used synonymously with CNFs but commonly refers to unmodified mechanically fibrillated cellulose composed of a heterogeneous mixture of nanoscale fibrils, thicker fibrils, and network-like structures, in contrast to NFC.
Micronucleus	A small extranuclear body formed from chromosome fragments or whole chromosomes not incorporated into daughter nuclei during cell division.
Micronucleus test in erythrocytes	A genotoxicity test evaluating chromosomal damage by measuring micronucleus formation in immature erythrocytes from bone marrow or peripheral blood.
Mouse lymphoma TK assay	A gene mutation assay using a mouse lymphoma cell line and the thymidine kinase (TK) gene as a marker for recessive mutations.
MWCNTs	Multi-walled carbon nanotubes.
Nanocellulose or nanocellulose materials (NCMs)	Cellulose-based materials with fiber diameters in the nanoscale range (approximately 1–100 nm), including CNFs and CNCs.
Nanocrystalline cellulose (NCC)	See cellulose nanocrystals (CNCs).
Nanofibrillated cellulose or nanofibrillar cellulose (NFC or NCF)	Often used synonymously with CNFs, but may indicate chemically modified CNFs with more uniform nanoscale fiber diameters, in contrast to MFC.
NEDO	New Energy and Industrial Technology Development Organization
NIOSH	National Institute for Occupational Safety and Health.
No observable adverse effect level (NOAEL)	The highest administered dose at which no adverse treatment-related effects are observed.
No observed effect concentration (NOEC)	The highest exposure concentration at which no statistically significant adverse effects are observed compared with controls in ecotoxicity tests.
OECD	Organisation for Economic Co-operation and Development.

OECD TG	OECD Test Guideline; internationally agreed testing methods for chemical safety evaluation, established and published by the OECD.
Optical particle counter (OPC)	An instrument that measures aerosol number concentration as a function of optical (light-scattering) particle diameter, typically in the range of approximately 0.3 to >10 μm (with lower limits depending on the model).
Oropharyngeal aspiration	An *in vivo* pulmonary exposure method in which a suspension of a test substance is placed in the pharynx of laboratory animals (e.g., rats or mice), resulting in aspiration into the lungs.
oxidative stress	A condition in which redox homeostasis shifts toward oxidation, potentially resulting in Biomolecular damage and disease, including carcinogenesis.
PEC	Predicted environmental concentration.
PNEC	Predicted no-effect concentration.
PSSD	Probabilistic species sensitivity distribution.
RCR	Risk characterization ratio; typically expressed as the ratio of PEC to PNEC and, in probabilistic assessments, informed by the overlap between their distributions.
Respirable dust	Dust collected using a size-selective sampler defined by ISO 7708, with a 50% collection efficiency for particles of 4 μm aerodynamic diameter.
ROS	Reactive oxygen species.
SEM	Scanning electron microscope.
SMPS	Scanning mobility particle sizer; an instrument that measures aerosol number concentration as a function of electrical mobility diameter, typically in the range of approximately 0.01–1 μm (with lower size limits down to ~0.001 μm, depending on the model).
TEM	Transmission electron microscope.
TEMPO	2,2,6,6-Tetramethylpiperidine 1-oxyl. TEMPO-oxidized CNFs are partially carboxylated through TEMPO-catalyzed oxidation.
TG	Test guideline.
UF	Uncertainty factor
USEPA	United States Environmental Protection Agency.

Chapter 1
Overview of the Book: Background, Scope, and Key Findings

Isamu Ogura and Katsuhide Fujita

Abstract This chapter presents an overview of the background, scope, structure, and principal findings of this book on the safety assessment of nanocellulose materials (NCMs), with a primary focus on cellulose nanofibrils (CNFs). The book is based on the outcomes of national research projects commissioned by the New Energy and Industrial Technology Development Organization (NEDO), together with an extensive review of the peer-reviewed literature. It integrates current scientific knowledge on human health hazards, exposure assessment, environmental impacts, and biodegradability of NCMs. This chapter outlines the conceptual framework of the book, clarifies terminology, and summarizes the key findings presented in each chapter.

Keywords Nanocellulose · Cellulose nanofibrils · Nanomaterial safety · Risk assessment · Safety assessment · Human health · Exposure assessment · Environmental impact · Biodegradability

1.1 Background and Rationale

Nanocellulose materials (NCMs)—including cellulose nanofibrils (CNFs) and cellulose nanocrystals (CNCs)—have attracted increasing industrial attention due to their sustainability, high strength-to-weight ratio, and strong applicability across diverse sectors. As bio-based materials derived from renewable resources such as wood, NCMs are expected to contribute to carbon-neutral societal transitions.

However, the unique physicochemical characteristics of industrial nanomaterials—such as extremely small size, high aspect ratio, surface reactivity, and agglomeration behavior—may lead to biological responses distinct from those of conventional chemicals. For the safe and widespread use of NCMs in society, it is

I. Ogura (✉) · K. Fujita
Research Institute of Science for Safety and Sustainability (RISS), National Institute of Advanced Industrial Science and Technology (AIST), Tsukuba, Ibaraki, Japan
e-mail: i-ogura@aist.go.jp; ka-fujita@aist.go.jp

I. Ogura, K. Fujita (eds.), *Nanocellulose Materials*,
https://doi.org/10.1007/978-981-92-2148-6_1

important to assess their safety in parallel with their development. The accumulation of safety information contributes to the sound development of the NCM industry, promotes appropriate voluntary safety management and application development by businesses, and enhances industrial competitiveness.

In response to this need, the National Institute of Advanced Industrial Science and Technology (AIST), in collaboration with industrial and academic partners, conducted two national research projects in Japan (FY2017–2019 and FY2020–2024), commissioned by the New Energy and Industrial Technology Development Organization (NEDO), aimed at establishing the scientific foundations for CNF safety assessment. These projects developed detection and quantification techniques, performed inhalation, dermal, oral, and ecotoxicity evaluations, and generated systematic exposure assessment data relevant to occupational settings. This book integrates these results with a comprehensive literature review to provide a consolidated scientific basis for evaluating NCM safety.

1.2 Materials Covered and Terminology

This book primarily focuses on CNFs (also referred to in the literature as cellulose nanofibers, CNFs; nanofibrillated cellulose, NFC; and microfibrillated cellulose, MFC), while also incorporating relevant information on CNCs and other NCMs. Conventional cellulose is used as a reference material where appropriate.

Terminology varies across publications; therefore, original terms are retained for contextual accuracy. The term NCMs is used as an overarching category throughout the book.

1.3 Structure of the Book

Chapters 2, 3, 4, 5, and 6 present findings on human health hazards, focusing on genotoxicity, mesothelioma, and route-specific effects (inhalation, dermal, and oral).

Chapter 7 addresses human exposure assessment and emission behavior.

Chapters 8 and 9 focus on ecological effects and biodegradability.

This integrated structure enables cross-referencing of hazard, exposure, and material properties, thereby supporting comprehensive risk assessment.

1.4 Key Findings

The key findings of this book are summarized below. These findings are based on an integrated evaluation of experimental results obtained in the NEDO projects and evidence from the peer-reviewed literature.

1.4.1 Human Health Impacts

1.4.1.1 Genotoxicity

Although some studies have reported DNA damage or genotoxic responses associated with NCMs under specific experimental conditions, well-established assays conducted in accordance with Organisation for Economic Co-operation and Development (OECD) test guidelines (TGs) have consistently yielded negative results. Consequently, no definitive conclusion has yet been reached regarding the genotoxic potential of NCMs. Under the NEDO projects, a comprehensive assessment was performed for three representative CNF types—TEMPO-oxidized, phosphorylated, and mechanically fibrillated—using a battery of OECD-compliant tests, including the Ames test, mouse lymphoma thymidine kinase (TK) assay, in vitro chromosomal aberration test, and rat erythrocyte micronucleus test. All evaluations were performed in strict compliance with OECD protocols, and all tested CNFs were consistently found to be negative for genotoxicity.

However, the physicochemical properties of NCMs—such as fiber length and diameter, surface functionalization, degree of fibrillation, crystallinity, and purity—can vary substantially depending on raw materials and manufacturing processes. This variability limits the generalizability of findings from any single study. Therefore, to ensure scientifically robust and internationally comparable safety evaluations, standardized genotoxicity test batteries should be conducted for each NCM type individually, following OECD TGs and employing fit-for-purpose approaches that account for material-specific characteristics.

1.4.1.2 Mesothelioma

In the NEDO project, three types of CNFs—mechanically fibrillated, TEMPO-oxidized, and phosphorylated CNFs—were administered intraperitoneally to mice and observed for a period of 2 years; however, no mesothelioma was detected in any of the CNF-treated groups. Although induction of chemokines and inflammatory cytokines was observed in the in vitro studies, no sustained inflammation was detected in the animal studies from 1 month after administration. Furthermore, no increase in inflammatory or mesothelioma-related biomarkers was observed throughout the study period, and no remarkable pathological findings attributable to CNF administration were identified. These findings suggest that the three types of CNFs are unlikely to induce sustained inflammation or mesothelioma in mesothelial tissue.

1.4.1.3 Inhalation Effects

Available evidence indicates that CNFs generally induce milder pulmonary inflammatory responses than CNCs and exhibit substantially less severe effects compared with carbon nanotubes (CNTs) or asbestos. However, the inhalation toxicity of

NCMs remains incompletely understood, particularly with respect to their persistence in lung tissue and potential long-term impacts. Intratracheal administration studies conducted under the NEDO projects demonstrated that CNFs can reach the alveoli and terminal bronchioles. Physical properties—such as fiber diameter and length—were found to influence deposition patterns and inflammatory responses in the lungs. Although CNF exposure induced mild acute pulmonary inflammation, these responses were resolved within 90 days and were substantially less pronounced than those observed following exposure to multiwalled CNTs under comparable conditions.

Nevertheless, CNFs may persist in lung tissue for extended periods, underscoring the need for comprehensive long-term evaluations that include endpoints beyond inflammation, such as fibrosis, genotoxicity, and systemic immune responses. In macrophage culture assays, CNFs were readily phagocytosed without inducing significant cytotoxicity, suggesting potential biocompatibility for certain NCM types. Importantly, variations in raw material sources and manufacturing processes substantially affect NCM physicochemical and biological properties—including fiber dimensions, surface chemistry, crystallinity, and endotoxin content—and must be carefully considered in biological impact assessments. Future research should systematically examine the relationship between NCM properties and biological responses across both in vitro and in vivo models and integrate findings across test systems to establish a comprehensive and reliable framework for inhalation safety evaluation.

1.4.1.4 Dermal Effects

Research on the dermal toxicity of NCMs remains limited; however, no adverse dermal effects have been reported to date. In the NEDO project, permeability testing using a three-dimensional reconstructed human skin model and fluorescently labeled TEMPO-oxidized CNFs demonstrated that CNFs did not penetrate the skin barrier and remained confined to the surface. This observation is consistent with existing literature indicating that substances with molecular weights exceeding approximately 500 Da are generally unlikely to permeate the stratum corneum. Accordingly, NCMs are considered to pose a low risk of transdermal absorption in healthy skin. Regarding skin irritation, TEMPO-oxidized CNFs were classified as nonirritant in a three-dimensional skin model test conducted in accordance with OECD TG 439. Similar outcomes have been reported in other studies using different skin models.

These findings alleviate concerns regarding dermal exposure to NCMs and demonstrate the value of advanced visualization techniques employed in this research. Future studies should address potential penetration through damaged or compromised skin barriers, as well as appendageal routes such as hair follicles and sweat glands. In addition, long-term and material-specific assessments remain necessary to account for variability in NCM physicochemical properties. Finally, the NEDO project confirmed the presence of common bacteria, fungi, endotoxins, and β-glucans in NCM suspensions. Endotoxins, even at trace amounts, exhibit strong biological activity and represent a critical safety concern for applications involving internal exposure, such as regenerative medicine and medical devices. Consequently, stringent quality control measures and contamination management strategies are essential to ensure the safe and responsible use of NCMs in biomedical applications.

1.4.1.5 Oral Toxicity

Reports on the oral toxicity of NCMs remain limited; however, existing studies consistently conclude that NCMs exhibit low toxicity. Furthermore, there is currently no evidence suggesting that NCMs are more hazardous than conventional cellulose.

Nevertheless, some studies have suggested that NCMs may reduce fat absorption, which could potentially lead to nutritional risks. Accordingly, additional studies are needed to include detailed evaluations of this effect, along with comprehensive long-term studies, to fully characterize the safety of NCMs in oral and dietary applications.

1.4.2 Human Exposure

For nanomaterials, inhalation exposure, especially in occupational environments, is widely regarded as a high-risk scenario; accordingly, most exposure assessment studies on NCMs have focused on airborne emissions and inhalation exposure.

Handling NCMs in dry powder form is associated with an increased likelihood of airborne particle release not only during routine operations but also during cleaning and maintenance; therefore, the use of local exhaust ventilation and appropriate personal protective equipment is recommended. Ventilation controls, including local exhaust systems such as fume hoods, have been shown to be effective in reducing airborne NCM concentrations.

In contrast, NCM aqueous suspensions are considerably less prone to aerosolization and are therefore less likely to become airborne or cause inhalation exposure compared with dry powders. In general, droplets larger than several tens of micrometers settle quickly due to gravity, while smaller droplets evaporate rapidly. Consequently, even when NCM-containing droplets are released into the air, inhalation exposure is expected to involve predominantly dry, densely aggregated particles, as smaller droplets rapidly evaporate. However, under conditions of very high humidity where droplet evaporation is suppressed, or when droplets consist of low-volatility liquids such as oils, exposure to dispersed NCMs may still occur.

During grinding or abrasion of CNF-containing composites, most airborne particles consist of resin fragments or resin–CNF mixtures. CNFs remain largely embedded within these particles, and direct exposure to isolated fibers is minimal. Therefore, effective control of resin dust emissions and exposure is expected to adequately manage CNF exposure.

1.4.3 Environmental Impacts

Overall, the impact of CNFs on aquatic organisms—including algae, crustaceans, and fish—is considered to be relatively low compared with that of typical chemical substances. Nevertheless, some studies have reported effects on algae even at the lowest tested concentration of 1 mg/L, indicating a need for additional data to clarify differences in algal responses depending on CNF type. In addition, chronic toxicity data for crustaceans and fish remain limited, and further research is necessary.

CNFs are prone to agglomeration and sedimentation in the presence of ions such as calcium and magnesium in environmental water, suggesting a tendency for CNFs to migrate from the water to sediments. Therefore, in addition to pelagic organisms such as algae, crustaceans, and fish, data on the effects of CNFs on benthic organisms are also needed.

Existing studies have rarely evaluated CNF concentrations and dispersion states in test solutions. To address this gap, the NEDO project established analytical methods for quantifying CNF concentrations and developed ecotoxicity testing protocols tailored to CNFs, taking into account dispersion stability and other factors. These methodological advances are expected to serve as valuable references for future ecotoxicity testing conducted by businesses.

Given the diversity of CNF physicochemical properties arising from differences in raw materials and manufacturing processes, toxicity may vary among CNF types. Accordingly, ecological impact assessment values—namely, predicted no-effect concentrations (PNECs)—should be derived for each CNF type, considering the extent of available data.

1.4.4 Biodegradability

Both CNFs and CNCs are generally considered biodegradable in a manner comparable to conventional cellulose. Although chemical modifications may affect biodegradability, general environmental biodegradation tests have shown that TEMPO-oxidized CNFs, phosphorylated CNFs, and acetylated CNFs are all readily biodegradable.

1.5 Important Notice

The findings presented in this book are based on specific types of NCMs and particular experimental conditions, and therefore cannot be generalized to all NCMs. Safety is determined by the combination of hazard and exposure, and a comprehensive risk assessment requires careful consideration of actual use conditions. Continued evaluation aligned with international standards—such as ISO Technical Reports and OECD Test Guidelines—is essential to ensure scientific validity and global comparability.

Chapter 2
Genotoxicity: Evidence, Mechanisms, and Safety Implications

Katsuhide Fujita

Abstract Genotoxicity assessment is essential for evaluating engineered nanomaterials, particularly fibrous nanoscale materials that may induce foreign-body-type responses in the lungs. Nanocellulose materials (NCMs)—including cellulose nanofibrils (CNFs, also referred to as cellulose nanofibers) and cellulose nanocrystals (CNCs)—are increasingly used across industrial and biomedical sectors, prompting examination of their potential genotoxic hazards. This chapter reviews published evidence together with findings from large-scale studies commissioned by the New Energy and Industrial Technology Development Organization (NEDO), emphasizing investigations conducted in accordance with OECD Test Guidelines to ensure high regulatory relevance. NCMs are also considered within the broader context of fibrous nanomaterial risk assessment, including comparisons with certain carbon nanotube types classified by the International Agency for Research on Cancer (IARC). Reported outcomes vary with surface chemistry, dimensions, additives, biological models, and assay design. Although some CNF formulations have shown localized DNA damage or oxidative-stress-related effects under specific conditions, OECD-compliant studies employing genotoxicity test batteries are predominantly negative. NEDO studies likewise reported consistently negative findings across assays for gene mutation and chromosomal damage. Overall, the available evidence indicates that the evaluated NCMs present a low genotoxic concern, while underscoring the importance of material-specific and exposure-relevant assessments.

Keywords Nanocellulose materials (NCMs) · Cellulose nanofibrils (CNFs) · Genotoxicity · DNA damage · Comet assay · Ames test · Mouse lymphoma TK assay · Micronucleus test · OECD Test Guideline

---

K. Fujita (✉)
Research Institute of Science for Safety and Sustainability (RISS), National Institute of Advanced Industrial Science and Technology (AIST), Tsukuba, Ibaraki, Japan
e-mail: ka-fujita@aist.go.jp

I. Ogura, K. Fujita (eds.), *Nanocellulose Materials*,
https://doi.org/10.1007/978-981-92-2148-6_2

2.1 Introduction

In the safety assessment of engineered nanomaterials, evaluation of genotoxic potential is a critical parameter for predicting and managing carcinogenic risks. This consideration is particularly important for materials with fibrous morphologies, which can trigger foreign-body-type responses in vivo. Such biological interactions highlight the need for early-stage evaluation and systematic risk assessment.

This chapter reviews current approaches to genotoxicity assessment of nanocellulose materials (NCMs), including cellulose nanofibrils (CNFs, also referred to as cellulose nanofibers) and cellulose nanocrystals (CNCs), and summarizes key findings from the NEDO-commissioned projects conducted during fiscal years 2017–2019 and 2020–2024.

Although NCMs are derived from renewable plant resources and are generally considered environmentally sustainable, their nanoscale dimensions and fibrous architectures have raised concerns regarding potential biological effects analogous to those observed with carbon nanotubes (CNTs), particularly with respect to carcinogenicity and genotoxicity. Consequently, systematic toxicological evaluation of NCMs is considered essential to ensure their safe and responsible use.

For fibrous engineered nanomaterials such as CNTs, which share certain morphological characteristics with asbestos, carcinogenic risks—most notably mesothelioma—have been a major global concern. Accordingly, extensive animal studies and exposure assessments have been conducted internationally. In 2016, Japan classified MWNT-7, a type of multi-walled carbon nanotube (MWCNT), under the carcinogenicity guidelines of the Industrial Safety and Health Act. Although MWNT-7 is no longer in production, the guidelines stipulate that products rebranded as "NT-7" or "NT-7K" must be handled as equivalent substances regardless of naming differences. In scientific literature and international reports, MWNT-7 is also referred to as MWCNT-7.

This regulatory action was informed in part by the 2014 classification by the International Agency for IARC, which categorized MWNT-7 as Group 2B (possibly carcinogenic to humans), while other CNTs were placed in Group 3 (not classifiable as to carcinogenicity in humans) (Grosse et al. 2014). In addition, research presented to a panel of the Ministry of Health, Labour and Welfare in 2015 reported the development of lung tumors in rats exposed to high concentrations of MWNT-7 over a 2-year period (Kasai et al. 2016). Although the implications for human health remain inconclusive, such findings reinforce the need for precautionary measures, including stringent exposure control and continued risk assessment.

Conversely, scientific data on the carcinogenicity and genotoxicity of other CNTs and nanocarbon materials remain limited, posing challenges for future regulatory frameworks and systematic risk evaluations. Likewise, scientific reports on the carcinogenic or genotoxic potential of NCMs remain limited. Considering their fibrous architectures and the likelihood of inhalation exposure, comprehensive evaluations—including controlled inhalation studies and biokinetic assessments—are warranted.

Carcinogenicity assessment of chemical substances typically involves long-term toxicity studies in rodents. For example, studies conducted in accordance with OECD Test Guidelines (TGs) 451 and 453 (OECD 2018a, b) require long-term exposure of test animals—via oral or inhalation routes—for up to 24 months, followed by histopathological examination to assess tumor incidence. Although scientifically robust, these methods are time-consuming and costly, limiting their routine use for broad chemical screening.

In recent years, international efforts to reduce or replace animal testing have accelerated the development and adoption of new approach methodologies (NAMs). Recent reports from the European Chemicals Agency (ECHA) highlight both the opportunities and remaining challenges in integrating NAMs into regulatory decision-making for industrial chemicals (ECHA 2023; Sewell et al. 2024).

Genotoxicity testing serves as an initial screening tool for carcinogenic potential and is widely employed due to its relative rapidity and cost-effectiveness. These assays detect genetic alterations—including DNA damage, chromosomal aberrations, micronucleus formation, and mutagenicity—using test systems broadly categorized as in vitro or in vivo.

OECD has promoted international harmonization of genotoxicity testing and, as of 2025, has established standardized test guidelines covering multiple assay types (https://doi.org/10.1787/20745788). These guidelines provide essential scientific evidence to support regulatory decision-making across jurisdictions.

Because individual assays capture only specific mechanisms of genotoxicity, relying on a single test provides an inherently incomplete assessment. Consequently, a battery approach employing multiple complementary assays is generally adopted. Regulatory frameworks—including the Industrial Safety and Health Act, the Chemical Substances Control Law, EU REACH, pharmaceutical regulations, and the Food Sanitation Act—specify combinations of tests tailored to their respective requirements. In pharmaceutical development, for example, a standard genotoxicity battery includes the Ames test, the mammalian cell chromosomal aberration test, and the in vivo micronucleus test in rodents (ICH S2(R1) 2012).

2.2 Information from Existing Literature

The genotoxicity of NCMs has been investigated across a variety of test systems and material types, yielding both positive and negative findings that reflect differences in physicochemical properties, study design, and assay endpoints. This section synthesizes representative studies to contextualize the current state of CNF genotoxicity assessment for an international readership.

Overall, several studies have reported positive genotoxicity outcomes—including DNA strand breaks and chromosomal alterations (de Lima et al. 2012; Catalán et al. 2017; Ventura et al. 2018; Hadrup et al. 2019; Aimonen et al. 2022; Vital et al. 2025) (Table 2.1). Among these, Catalán et al. (2017) explicitly reported compliance with OECD TG 489 (OECD 2016c) and TG 471 (OECD 2020), demonstrating DNA damage in murine lung cells following pharyngeal aspiration of CNFs.

Table 2.1 Summary of published studies evaluating the genotoxicity of nanocellulose materials (NCMs)

Test material	Cells/Animals	Test method	Test results	References
TEMPO-oxidized CNFs	A549 (co-cultured with THP-1)	Comet assay, micronucleus test	No DNA damage detected in the comet assay; increased micronucleus formation observed at 1.5 and 3 μg/cm², suggesting potential chromosomal damage	Ventura et al. (2018)
TEMPO-oxidized CNFs, CMFs, CNCs	A549 (co-cultured with THP-1)	Comet assay, micronucleus test	CNFs and CNCs showed no genotoxicity in comet assay; CMFs induced DNA strand breaks in the comet assay at the lowest tested concentration. No chromosomal abnormalities observed in micronucleus test for all materials	Ventura et al. (2023)
TEMPO-oxidized CNFs	Lung cells and BAL cells	Comet assay, bone marrow micronucleus test (OECD TG 489, TG 471)	DNA damage observed in lung cells at low doses; no DNA damage detected in BAL cells and no micronucleus induction in bone marrow	Catalán et al. (2017)
CNFs, Carboxylated CNFs	Mice via intratracheal instillation	Comet assay	DNA damage observed in BAL cells and lung tissue, with responses varying by CNF type and exposure duration	Hadrup et al. (2019)
CNFs from cotton and curaua fibers	Onion root, human lymphocytes, mouse fibroblasts	Chromosomal aberration test, comet assay	Source-dependent DNA damage observed. Brown cotton and curaua CNFs induced genotoxic effects in plant and animal cells, whereas ruby cotton CNFs showed no DNA damage	de Lima et al. (2012)

(continued)

Table 2.1 (continued)

Test material	Cells/Animals	Test method	Test results	References
Unmodified CNFs, TEMPO-CNFs, EPTMAC-CNFs, CMC-CNFs, Raw fibers	BEAS-2B cells	Comet assay, micronucleus test	DNA strand breaks and/or chromosomal damage observed in fine EPTMAC-CNFs and coarse CMC-CNFs; no genotoxic effects detected in other CNF fractions or raw fibers	Aimonen et al. (2022)
TEMPO-CNFs, Enzymatically degraded CNFs	Caco-2 and HT29-MTX-E12 cells	Comet assay, micronucleus test (OECD TG 487)	Negative for gene mutation and chromosomal damage endpoints; DNA damage was observed in comet assays. Digested TEMPO-oxidized CNFs yielded an equivocal micronucleus response at the lowest tested concentration	Vital et al. (2025)
CNFs from banana pseudostem	Caco-2 cells	Comet assay	No DNA damage detected in the comet assay; no adverse findings in repeated-dose oral studies	Mejía-Jaramillo et al. (2023)
Finely ground fibrillated cellulose	*Salmonella* spp., *E. coli*	Ames test (OECD TG 471)	Negative in the Ames test and in vivo genotoxicity assays	Pitkänen et al. (2014)
Bacterial cellulose nanofiber	CHO cells, *Salmonella* spp., *E. coli*	Ames test, comet assay (OECD TG 471, TG 489)	Negative in both Ames and comet assays	Moreira et al. (2009)
CNCs, Microcrystalline cellulose	BEAS-2B cells	Micronucleus test (OECD TG 487)	CNCs: Negative in micronucleus assay; MCC induced inflammatory cytokine responses but showed no genotoxic effects	Catalán et al. (2015)
CNFs from cedar pulp	*Salmonella* spp., *E. coli*, CHL/IU cells	Ames test, chromosomal aberration test (OECD TG 471, TG 473)	Negative in Ames and chromosomal aberration assays	Shimokawa et al. (2021a)
CNFs from bamboo pulp	*Salmonella* spp., *E. coli*, mouse lymphoma cells, CHL/IU cells	Ames test, mouse lymphoma TK test, micronucleus test (OECD TG 471, TG 490, TG 487)	No evidence of gene mutation or chromosomal damage across all tested endpoints	Shimokawa et al. (2021b)

(continued)

Table 2.1 (continued)

Test material	Cells/Animals	Test method	Test results	References
TEMPO-CNFs, Phosphorylated CNFs, Mechanically fibrillated CNFs	*Salmonella* spp., *E. coli*, mouse lymphoma cells, CHL/IU cells, rat blood cells	Ames test, mouse lymphoma TK test, chromosomal aberration test, rat micronucleus test (OECD TG 471, TG 490, TG 473, TG 474)	Negative across assays for gene mutation and chromosomal damage, including Ames, mouse lymphoma TK, chromosomal aberration, and rat micronucleus tests	Fujita et al. (2021)

In contrast, numerous studies have reported negative genotoxicity findings. For example, Mejía-Jaramillo et al. (2023) observed no DNA damage in a comet assay using human Caco-2 cells. Importantly, many studies reporting negative results were conducted in accordance with the OECD TGs (Moreira et al. 2009; Pitkänen et al. 2014; Catalán et al. 2015; Shimokawa et al. 2021a, b; Fujita et al. 2021), thereby strengthening the credibility and regulatory relevance of their conclusions.

Notably, battery-testing studies by Shimokawa et al. (2021b) and Fujita et al. (2021) employed multiple in vitro genotoxicity assays and consistently reported negative outcomes across platforms. These results provide convergent evidence supporting the absence of genotoxic effects under the tested conditions. Detailed outcomes from Fujita et al. (2021) are presented in Sect. 2.3.

Terminology Note

Some cited studies refer to nanofibrillated cellulose as NFC or NCF. For consistency, this chapter uses the term CNF to describe these materials collectively.

2.2.1 Study Summaries

Ventura et al. (2018) evaluated TEMPO-oxidized CNFs from *Eucalyptus globulus* kraft pulp using a human alveolar coculture model (A549 epithelial cells with THP-1 macrophages). Low CNF concentrations enhanced A549 proliferation, whereas higher concentrations produced moderate cytotoxicity. IL-1β remained undetectable under coculture conditions, indicating minimal immunotoxicity. While comet assays showed no DNA damage, micronucleus assays revealed increased micronuclei at 1.5 and 3 μg/cm^2, suggesting potential aneugenic or clastogenic effects. Collectively, the results underscore the need for formulation- and dose-specific safety evaluations.

Building on this work, Ventura et al. (2023) assessed the genotoxicity of cellulose micro- and nanomaterials (CMNMs), including cellulose microfibrils (CMFs), CNFs, and cellulose nanocrystals (CNCs), all derived from *E. globulus*. Using the same coculture model and a combination of comet assays (including FPG-modified comet assays for oxidative DNA lesions) and micronucleus tests, DNA strand breaks were observed only at the lowest CMF concentration. CNFs and CNCs did not induce chromosomal alterations. Collectively, these studies suggest that TEMPO-oxidized CNFs and CNCs are nongenotoxic under the tested conditions, whereas CMFs may exhibit low genotoxic potential.

Catalán et al. (2017) evaluated the genotoxic and inflammatory effects of TEMPO-oxidized CNFs in female C57BL/6 mice following single pharyngeal aspiration dose ranging from 10 to 200 μg per mouse. DNA damage was observed in lung cells at lower doses, while no increase was detected in the bronchoalveolar lavage (BAL) cell counts. Bone marrow micronucleus assays were negative, indicating no systemic genotoxicity. CNF exposure induced dose-dependent increases in lung mRNA expression of TNF-α, IL-1β, IL-6, and CXCL5, although corresponding protein levels remained largely unchanged. Histological analysis revealed dose-dependent CNF accumulation, macrophage uptake, and neutrophil infiltration in alveolar regions, supporting the conclusion that CNFs induce acute, localized pulmonary inflammation and lung DNA damage without systemic genotoxicity.

Hadrup et al. (2019) examined three CNF types—FINE CNF, carboxylated CNF (AS–COOH), and biocide-containing CNF (BIOCID FINE CNF)—administered to mice via intratracheal instillation. FINE CNF induced lung DNA damage 1 day after exposure, while AS–COOH CNF caused DNA damage in BAL cells at 28 days in the highest dose group. BIOCID FINE CNF produced higher DNA damage than FINE CNF, implicating biocide contributions to the observed effects.

de Lima et al. (2012) evaluated CNFs derived from agricultural sources (brown cotton, curaua, and ruby cotton) using onion root cells and cultured human lymphocytes and fibroblasts. Source- and cell-type-specific DNA damage was observed: CNFs from brown cotton and curaua were genotoxic in both models, whereas ruby cotton CNFs did not induce DNA damage. These findings emphasize the importance of source-specific safety assessments.

Aimonen et al. (2022) investigated CNFs differing in surface chemistry (unmodified, TEMPO-oxidized, carboxymethylated, and cationic) and size fraction (fine, medium, and coarse) in bronchial epithelial BEAS-2B cells. Most CNFs increased reactive oxygen species (ROS) production. Fine cationic CNFs induced DNA strand breaks and chromosomal damage, while coarse carboxymethylated CNFs caused chromosomal alterations. These results implicate oxidative stress as a key mechanism and reinforce the need for formulation-specific evaluations.

Vital et al. (2025) assessed two NCMs—TEMPO-oxidized CNFs and enzymatically processed CMFs—using human intestinal Caco-2 cells under in vitro digestion conditions and genotoxicity battery tests. No gene mutations or chromosomal alterations were detected across standard endpoints; however, comet assays indicated DNA strand breaks, suggesting possible genotoxicity. Digested CNFs generally showed reduced DNA damage, although the lowest concentration of digested TEMPO-oxidized CNFs yielded an equivocal micronucleus response. These findings suggest that while the initial results are largely reassuring, the genotoxic potential cannot be fully excluded, warranting further investigation including epigenotoxic mechanisms for food-related applications.

Mejía-Jaramillo et al. (2023) evaluated banana rachis-derived CNFs intended for food packaging and functional ingredient applications. In Caco-2 cells, no cytotoxicity or DNA damage was observed in comet assays. In vivo studies involving single and repeated oral dosing over 1 month revealed no pathological changes in liver, kidney, or intestinal tissues, and histological and biochemical parameters remained within normal ranges, supporting a nontoxic and nongenotoxic profile under the tested conditions.

Pitkänen et al. (2014) examined the relationship between size fractionation of fibrillated cellulose and toxicity. Slight cytotoxicity was observed at the highest concentrations, but Ames tests and in vivo nematode assays indicated no genotoxicity. The potential influence of biocides used during material preparation was identified as an important area for further investigation.

Moreira et al. (2009) reported that bacterial cellulose nanofibers produced via acid hydrolysis and ultrasonic treatment were nongenotoxic in both comet and Ames assays. Although a slight reduction in fibroblast and CHO cell proliferation was observed, no morphological changes occurred, supporting low cytotoxicity and genotoxic safety under the tested conditions.

Catalán et al. (2015) compared CNCs with microcrystalline cellulose (MCC) as a non-nanoscale reference in BEAS-2B cells. Both materials exhibited cytotoxicity at 100 μg/mL, but no micronucleus formation was observed, indicating no genotoxicity. In macrophages, MCC induced pro-inflammatory cytokine release following LPS priming, whereas CNCs did not. These findings underscore the importance of distinguishing nanoscale from non-nanoscale cellulose in safety assessments and highlight the need for further in vivo studies addressing inflammation-mediated genotoxicity.

Shimokawa et al. (2021a) conducted Ames and chromosomal aberration assays using cedar pulp-derived CNFs, yielding negative results for genotoxicity. Shimokawa et al. (2021b) evaluated bamboo pulp-derived CNFs using a comprehensive in vitro test battery—including Ames, mouse lymphoma thymidine kinase (TK), and micronucleus assays—and reported no evidence of gene mutations or chromosomal damage across all systems.

Finally, Joint FAO/WHO Expert Committee on Food Additives (JECFA) (1998) reviewed MCC used as a food additive and reported negative results in Ames, mouse lymphoma TK, and micronucleus assays, collectively supporting the genotoxic safety of MCC under typical use conditions.

2.2.2 Synthesis and Implications

Taken together, the literature demonstrates heterogeneous outcomes influenced by material characteristics (e.g., surface chemistry, size fraction, presence of additives/biocides), biological models, and assay selection. Studies conducted in accordance with OECD TGs and battery approaches offer greater regulatory confidence, particularly where concordant negative results are observed (e.g., Shimokawa et al.

2021b; Fujita et al. 2021). Nevertheless, evidence of localized pulmonary DNA damage and oxidative stress-mediated mechanisms for certain CNF formulations (e.g., TEMPO-oxidized and cationic) suggest that formulation-specific and exposure-relevant evaluations remain essential. Consistent with the precautionary framework outlined in Sect. 2.1, these findings support a risk-based approach that integrates physicochemical profiling, fit-for-purpose test batteries, and targeted in vivo follow-up for signals arising from in vitro assays, where applicable. This approach aligns with historical safety evaluations, such as those by JECFA (1998) for MCC safety in food applications, reinforcing the importance of context-specific risk assessment for emerging NCMs.

2.3 Key Findings from the NEDO Project

Comprehensive genotoxicity battery testing has previously been applied to engineered nanomaterials, including MWCNTs and exfoliated graphene (Ema et al. 2012; Fujita et al. 2018). Building on this established framework, the NEDO projects conducted during fiscal years 2017–2019 and 2020–2024 systematically evaluated the genotoxic potential of NCMs using internationally recognized testing strategies.

The evaluation employed a standardized battery of four OECD-compliant assays: the bacterial reverse mutation (Ames) test, the mouse lymphoma TK assay, the in vitro chromosomal aberration test, and the rat erythrocyte micronucleus test (Fujita et al. 2023) (Fig. 2.1). This integrated approach enabled a comprehensive assessment of both gene mutation and chromosomal damage, allowing for robust

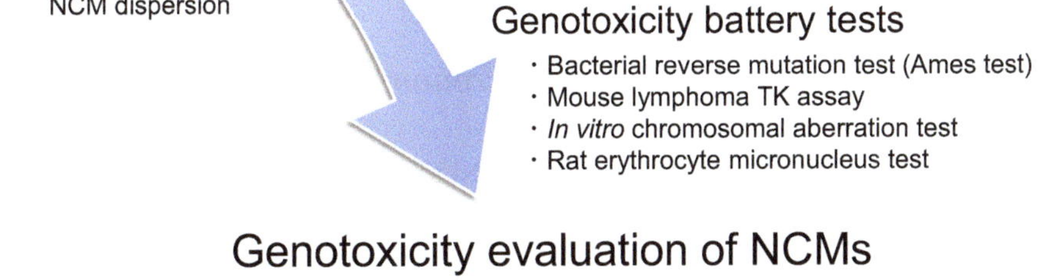

Fig. 2.1 Integrated genotoxicity evaluation of nanocellulose materials (NCMs) using a battery of four OECD-compliant assays

cross-material comparisons while ensuring alignment with international regulatory expectations.

2.3.1 Ames Test (OECD TG 471)

Three types of NCMs—phosphorylated CNFs, TEMPO-oxidized CNFs, and mechanically fibrillated CNFs—were assessed for mutagenicity using *Salmonella typhimurium* strains TA100, TA1535, TA98, and TA1537, as well as *Escherichia coli* WP2uvrA, in accordance with OECD TG 471 (OECD 2020). Tests were conducted both in the presence (+S9) and absence (–S9) of metabolic activation. Across six dose levels up to 100 µg/plate, none of the tested NCMs produced revertant colony numbers exceeding twice those of the negative control. All positive controls elicited clear mutagenic responses, confirming assay validity. Accordingly, all tested NCMs were evaluated as negative for mutagenicity under the conditions employed.

2.3.2 Mouse Lymphoma TK Assay (OECD TG 490)

Although the Ames test remains an internationally accepted component of standard genotoxicity testing batteries, mammalian cell gene mutation assays are generally recommended for engineered nanomaterials because the utility of the Ames test is considered limited (Landsiedel et al. 2009, 2022; Elespuru et al. 2018). Accordingly, mutation testing was performed using L5178Y tk± mouse lymphoma cells in accordance with OECD TG 490 (OECD 2016d). TEMPO-oxidized CNFs and mechanically fibrillated CNFs were examined under three exposure conditions: short-term treatment with metabolic activation (+S9), short-term treatment without activation (–S9), and 24-h continuous treatment without activation. At concentrations up to 100 µg/mL, mutation frequencies remained below the global evaluation factor under all exposure conditions. Positive controls induced the expected increases in mutation frequency, validating assay performance. Both CNFs were therefore judged to be negative for gene mutation induction.

2.3.3 In vitro Chromosomal Aberration Test (OECD TG 473)

Phosphorylated CNFs, TEMPO-oxidized CNFs, and mechanically fibrillated CNFs were evaluated for their potential to induce structural chromosomal aberrations and polyploidy in CHL/IU cells, in accordance with OECD TG 473 (OECD 2016a). No statistically significant increases in aberrant cells or polyploid cells were observed at concentrations up to 100 µg/mL. The responsiveness of the test system was confirmed by positive controls, including mitomycin C and cyclophosphamide. Based on these results, all tested NCMs were considered negative for chromosomal aberration induction.

2.3.4 Rat Erythrocyte Micronucleus Test (OECD TG 474)

In vivo genotoxic potential was assessed using a rat bone marrow micronucleus test, in accordance with OECD TG 474 (OECD 2016b). The same three NCMs were administered by intratracheal instillation at doses of 0.5, 1.0, and 2.0 mg/kg/day for two consecutive days. Micronucleated polychromatic erythrocytes (MNPCEs) and the ratio of polychromatic erythrocytes were evaluated. No statistically significant increases in MNPCE frequency or alterations in erythrocyte ratios were observed in any treatment group. Positive controls produced the expected responses, confirming assay reliability. All tested NCMs were therefore judged to be negative for micronucleus induction in vivo.

2.3.5 Integrated Genotoxicity Evaluation

Taken together, the results from the four OECD-compliant genotoxicity assays indicate that phosphorylated CNFs, TEMPO-oxidized CNFs, and mechanically fibrillated CNFs did not exhibit genotoxic effects under the tested conditions and were evaluated as negative across all endpoints (Fujita et al. 2021). These findings provide robust evidence that, within the scope of standardized genotoxicity testing, the tested NCMs present a low genotoxic concern. Nonetheless, given the wide diversity in physicochemical properties among NCMs—including differences in morphology, dimensions, surface chemistry, and manufacturing processes—case-by-case evaluation remains essential for comprehensive safety assessment.

2.4 Summary

This chapter integrates evidence from the published literature with results obtained from standardized genotoxicity testing to summarize the current understanding of the genotoxic potential of NCMs. Although some studies have reported DNA damage or genotoxic responses under specific experimental conditions, outcomes derived from OECD guideline-compliant assays have been predominantly negative. Consequently, a definitive consensus on the genotoxic potential of NCMs has not yet been established. The variability in reported outcomes appears to be associated with differences in physicochemical properties (e.g., dimensions and surface chemistry), as well as the presence of additives and variations in biological models and experimental design.

In contrast, the comprehensive battery of genotoxicity assays conducted within the NEDO projects—including the Ames test, mouse lymphoma TK assay, in vitro chromosomal aberration test, and rat erythrocyte micronucleus test—consistently yielded negative results for phosphorylated CNFs, TEMPO-oxidized CNFs, and mechanically fibrillated CNFs. These findings are consistent with the overall trend observed in OECD guideline-compliant studies and further support a low genotoxic concern under conditions relevant to standard regulatory testing.

Collectively, these findings indicate that the tested NCMs did not exhibit genotoxic effects under the conditions evaluated. Nevertheless, given the substantial variability in physicochemical properties among NCMs—such as fiber length and diameter, morphology, surface functionalization, degree of fibrillation, and material purity—arising from differences in raw materials and manufacturing processes, material-specific, OECD-compliant evaluations remain essential to ensure reliable and context-appropriate safety assessments.

References

Aimonen K, Imani M, Hartikainen M, Suhonen S, Vanhala E, Moreno C, Rojas OJ, Norppa H, Catalán J (2022) Surface functionalization and size modulate the formation of reactive oxygen species and genotoxic effects of cellulose nanofibrils. Part Fibre Toxicol 19(1):19. https://doi.org/10.1186/s12989-022-00460-3

Catalán J, Ilves M, Järventaus H, Hannukainen KS, Kontturi E, Vanhala E, Alenius H, Savolainen KM, Norppa H (2015) Genotoxic and immunotoxic effects of cellulose nanocrystals in vitro. Environ Mol Mutagen 56(2):171–182. https://doi.org/10.1002/em.21913

Catalán J, Rydman E, Aimonen K, Hannukainen KS, Suhonen S, Vanhala E, Moreno C, Meyer V, Perez DD, Sneck A, Forsström U, Højgaard C, Willemoes M, Winther JR, Vogel U, Wolff H, Alenius H, Savolainen KM, Norppa H (2017) Genotoxic and inflammatory effects of nanofibrillated cellulose in murine lungs. Mutagenesis 32(1):23–31. https://doi.org/10.1093/mutage/gew035

de Lima R, Oliveira Feitosa L, Rodrigues Maruyama C, Abreu Barga M, Yamawaki PC, Vieira IJ, Teixeira EM, Corrêa AC, Caparelli Mattoso LH, Fernandes Fraceto L (2012) Evaluation of the genotoxicity of cellulose nanofibers. Int J Nanomedicine 7:3555–3565. https://doi.org/10.2147/IJN.S30596

ECHA, European Chemicals Agency (2023) Report on the European Chemicals Agency's "new approach methodologies workshop: towards an animal-free regulatory system for industrial chemicals". En: European Union, Helsinki, Finland, Brussels. ECHA-23-R-09 ISBN: 978-92-9468-299-4. Cat. No.: ED-04-23-926-EN-N, p 2023. https://doi.org/10.2823/7494

Elespuru R, Pfuhler S, Aardema MJ, Chen T, Doak SH, Doherty A, Farabaugh CS, Kenny J, Manjanatha M, Mahadevan B, Moore MM, Ouédraogo G, Stankowski LF Jr, Tanir JY (2018) Genotoxicity assessment of nanomaterials: recommendations on best practices, assays, and methods. Toxicol Sci 164(2):391–416. https://doi.org/10.1093/toxsci/kfy100

Ema M, Imamura T, Suzuki H, Kobayashi N, Naya M, Nakanishi J (2012) Evaluation of genotoxicity of multi-walled carbon nanotubes in a battery of in vitro and in vivo assays. Regul Toxicol Pharmacol 63(2):188–195. https://doi.org/10.1016/j.yrtph.2012.03.014

Fujita K, Take S, Tani R, Maru J, Obara S, Endoh S (2018) Assessment of cytotoxicity and mutagenicity of exfoliated graphene. Toxicol in Vitro 52:195–202. https://doi.org/10.1016/j.tiv.2018.06.016

Fujita K, Obara S, Maru J, Endoh S (2021) Genotoxicity assessment of cellulose nanofibrils using a standard battery of in vitro and in vivo assays. Toxicol Rep 9:68–77. https://doi.org/10.1016/j.toxrep.2021.12.006

Fujita K, Endoh S, Maru J, Sai T, Tomoko A, Goi Y, Obara S, Tani F, Yamamoto F, Ogawa T (2023) A manual for toxicity testing of cellulose nanofibers. https://riss.aist.go.jp/results-and-dissemin/776/

Grosse Y, Loomis D, Guyton KZ, Lauby-Secretan B, El Ghissassi F, Bouvard V, Benbrahim-Tallaa L, Guha N, Scoccianti C, Mattock H, Straif K, International Agency for Research on Cancer Monograph Working Group (2014) Carcinogenicity of fluoro-edenite, silicon carbide fibres and whiskers, and carbon nanotubes. Lancet Oncol 15(13):1427–1428. https://doi.org/10.1016/S1470-2045(14)71109-X

Hadrup N, Knudsen KB, Berthing T, Wolff H, Bengtson S, Kofoed C, Espersen R, Højgaard C, Winther JR, Willemoës M, Wedin I, Nuopponen M, Alenius H, Norppa H, Wallin H, Vogel U (2019) Pulmonary effects of nanofibrillated celluloses in mice suggest that carboxylation lowers the inflammatory and acute phase responses. Environ Toxicol Pharmacol 66:116–125. https://doi.org/10.1016/j.etap.2019.01.003

ICH S2(R1) (2012) Genotoxicity testing and data interpretation for pharmaceuticals intended for human use—scientific guideline. European Medicines Agency (EMA) Adopted June 2012. https://www.ema.europa.eu/en/ich-s2-r1-genotoxicity-testing-data-interpretation-pharmaceuticals-intended-human-use-scientific-guideline

Joint FAO/WHO Expert Committee on Food Additives (JECFA) (1998) Safety evaluation of certain food additives and contaminants. WHO Food Addit S 40. Microcrystalline cellulose. https://inchem.org/documents/jecfa/jecmono/v040je03.htm

Kasai T, Umeda Y, Ohnishi M, Mine T, Kondo H, Takeuchi T, Matsumoto M, Fukushima S (2016) Lung carcinogenicity of inhaled multi-walled carbon nanotube in rats. Part Fibre Toxicol 13(1):53. https://doi.org/10.1186/s12989-016-0164-2

Landsiedel R, Kapp MD, Schulz M, Wiench K, Oesch F (2009) Genotoxicity investigations on nanomaterials: methods, preparation and characterization of test material, potential artifacts and limitations—many questions, some answers. Mutat Res 681(2–3):241–258. https://doi.org/10.1016/j.mrrev.2008.10.002

Landsiedel R, Honarvar N, Seiffert SB, Oesch B, Oesch F (2022) Genotoxicity testing of nanomaterials. Wiley Interdiscip Rev Nanomed Nanobiotechnol 14(6):e1833. https://doi.org/10.1002/wnan.1833

Mejía-Jaramillo AM, Gómez-Hoyos C, Cañas Gutierrez AI, Correa-Hincapié N, Zuluaga Gallego R, Triana-Chávez O (2023) Tackling the cytotoxicity and genotoxicity of cellulose nanofibers from the banana rachis: a new food packaging alternative. Heliyon 9(11):e2(1560). https://doi.org/10.1016/j.heliyon.2023.e21560

Moreira S, Silva NB, Almeida-Lima J, Rocha HAO, Medeiros SRB, Alves C Jr, Gama FM (2009) BC nanofibres: in vitro study of genotoxicity and cell proliferation. Toxicol Lett 189(3):235–241. https://doi.org/10.1016/j.toxlet.2009.06.849

OECD (2016a) Test no. 473: in vitro mammalian chromosomal aberration test, OECD guidelines for the testing of chemicals, section 4. OECD Publishing, Paris. https://doi.org/10.1787/9789264264649-en

OECD (2016b) Test no. 474: mammalian erythrocyte micronucleus test, OECD guidelines for the testing of chemicals, section 4. OECD Publishing, Paris. https://doi.org/10.1787/9789264264762-en

OECD (2016c) Test no. 489: in vivo mammalian alkaline comet assay, OECD guidelines for the testing of chemicals, section 4. OECD Publishing, Paris. https://doi.org/10.1787/9789264264885-en

OECD (2016d) Test no. 490: in vitro mammalian cell gene mutation tests using the thymidine kinase gene, OECD guidelines for the testing of chemicals, section 4. OECD Publishing, Paris. https://doi.org/10.1787/9789264264908-en

OECD (2018a) Test no. 451: carcinogenicity studies, OECD guidelines for the testing of chemicals, section 4. OECD Publishing, Paris. https://doi.org/10.1787/9789264071186-en

OECD (2018b) Test no. 453: combined chronic toxicity/carcinogenicity studies, OECD guidelines for the testing of chemicals, section 4. OECD Publishing, Paris. https://doi.org/10.1787/9789264071223-en

OECD (2020) Test no. 471: bacterial reverse mutation test, OECD guidelines for the testing of chemicals, section 4. OECD Publishing, Paris. https://doi.org/10.1787/9789264071247-en

Pitkänen M, Kangas H, Laitinen O, Sneck A, Lahtinen P, Peresin MS, Niinimäki J (2014) Characteristics and safety of nano-sized cellulose fibrils. Cellulose 21(6):3871–3886. https://doi.org/10.1007/s10570-014-0397-x

Sewell F, Alexander-White C, Brescia S, Currie RA, Roberts R, Roper C, Vickers C, Westmoreland C, Kimber I (2024) New approach methodologies (NAMs): identifying and overcoming hurdles to accelerated adoption. Toxicol Res (Camb) 13(2):tfae044. https://doi.org/10.1093/toxres/tfae044

Shimokawa T, Magara K, Nojiri M, Hayashi N (2021a) Safety evaluation of cellulose nanofibers produced from soda–anthraquinone sugi pulp by enzymatic treatment and wet milling. Jpn Tappi J 75(8):757–764. (in Japanese)

Shimokawa T, Magara K, Ikeda T, Hayashi N, Ogawa M, Takao T, Nakayama E (2021b) Safety assessment of cellulose nanofibers obtained from soda cooking bamboo pulp: bacterial reverse mutation test, mouse lymphoma thymidine kinase assay, micronucleus test, and repeated dose 90-day oral administration in rats. Jpn Tappi J 75(11):1034–1050. https://doi.org/10.2524/jtappij.75.1034

Ventura C, Lourenço AF, Sousa-Uva A, Ferreira PJT, Silva MJ (2018) Evaluating the genotoxicity of cellulose nanofibrils in a co-culture of human lung epithelial cells and monocyte-derived macrophages. Toxicol Lett 291:173–183. https://doi.org/10.1016/j.toxlet.2018.04.013

Ventura C, Pinto F, Lourenço AF, Pedrosa JFS, Fernandes SN, da Rosa RR, Godinho MH, Ferreira PJT, Louro H, Silva MJ (2023) Assessing the genotoxicity of cellulose nanomaterials in a co-culture of human lung epithelial cells and monocyte-derived macrophages. Bioengineering (Basel) 10(8):986. https://doi.org/10.3390/bioengineering10080986

Vital N, Cardoso M, Kranendonk M, Silva MJ, Louro H (2025) Evaluation of the cyto- and genotoxicity of two types of cellulose nanomaterials using human intestinal cells and in vitro digestion simulation. Arch Toxicol 99(2):575–596. https://doi.org/10.1007/s00204-024-03911-2

Chapter 3
Mesothelioma Potential: Comparative Insights and Safety Findings

Masanori Horie

Abstract Fibrous nanomaterials raise concerns regarding the potential risk of mesothelioma following inhalation exposure, analogous to asbestos; however, the mesothelioma-inducing potential of nanocellulose materials remains unclear. This chapter first provides an overview of mesothelioma and mesothelial cell-related biological responses induced by asbestos and multiwalled carbon nanotubes, based on existing studies. Proposed mechanisms include oxidative stress induction, disruption of cell division, and adsorption of harmful substances. Phagocytosis by mesothelial cells, long-term retention, and the influence of fiber morphology, rigidity, and iron contamination are also considered critical factors. This chapter then presents findings from the NEDO project evaluating the mesothelioma-inducing potential of cellulose nanofibrils (CNFs; also called cellulose nanofibers) using long-term intraperitoneal administration in mice and complementary in vitro assays with mesothelial cells and macrophages. Three CNF types—mechanically fibrillated, TEMPO-oxidized, and phosphorylated—were administered and observed for 2 years; no mesothelioma was detected in any CNF-treated group. Although chemokine and inflammatory cytokine induction was observed in macrophages in vitro, no sustained inflammation occurred in vivo after 1 month, inflammatory and mesothelioma-related biomarkers did not increase, and no notable CNF-related pathological changes were observed. These findings suggest that the three types of CNFs are unlikely to induce sustained inflammation or mesothelioma.

Keywords Nanocellulose · Cellulose nanofibrils · Methothelioma · Mesothelin · Osteopontin · Inflammation · Intratracheal instillation

---

M. Horie (✉)
Health and Medical Research Institute, National Institute of Advanced Industrial Science and Technology (AIST), Takamatsu, Kagawa, Japan
e-mail: masa-horie@aist.go.jp

I. Ogura, K. Fujita (eds.), *Nanocellulose Materials*,
https://doi.org/10.1007/978-981-92-2148-6_3

3.1 Introduction

Fibrous nanomaterials raise concerns regarding the potential risk of mesothelioma following inhalation exposure, analogous to asbestos. To date, however, no studies have verified the development of mesothelioma caused by nanocellulose materials (NCMs), and their potential to induce mesothelioma remains unclear. Scientific evaluation of the plausibility of mesothelioma induction by NCMs is therefore important for ensuring occupational health and safety and for supporting their practical application.

Mesothelioma is a malignant tumor arising from mesothelial cells and is considered a rare cancer. The majority of documented cases have been linked to asbestos inhalation (Chen et al. 2024). Mesothelioma occurs at sites lined by mesothelial cells, including the pleura, peritoneum, pericardium, and tunica vaginalis of the testis. Among these, pleural mesothelioma accounts for 80–90% of cases due to frequent exposure of the pleura to harmful substances via the respiratory tract, followed by peritoneal mesothelioma, which accounts for approximately 10% of cases (Inai et al. 2007).

A commonly used method to evaluate the potential for mesothelioma induction is the intraperitoneal administration test, in which a test substance is administered into the peritoneal cavity of rodents and tumor formation in peritoneal mesothelial cells is assessed. This method has been widely employed in studies of asbestos and multiwalled carbon nanotubes (MWCNTs). Considering the anatomical sites of mesothelioma occurrence, evaluation of pleural mesothelioma induction via intratracheal administration of the test substance is effective as it mimics the actual exposure route. However, intratracheal intubation and administration require technical expertise, and when performed by inexperienced operators, uneven distribution of the test substance in the lungs may occur. Strict technical control of the administered dose is therefore necessary. In addition, limitations include the relatively small volumes of biological samples obtainable—such as bronchoalveolar lavage fluid—which can restrict the range of measurable biomarkers. In contrast, intraperitoneal administration enables easier control of the administered dose and allows collection of larger volumes of biological samples. This facilitates evaluation of the potential for mesothelioma induction by the test substance and enables more extensive mechanistic analyses of tumor development if mesothelioma occurs. Consequently, intraperitoneal administration has been widely adopted in experimental mesothelioma studies.

This chapter provides an overview of mesothelioma and mesothelial cell–related biological responses induced by asbestos and MWCNTs, based on existing studies. It also presents findings from the NEDO project (FY2020–2024) evaluating the mesothelioma induction potential of cellulose nanofibrils (also referred to as cellulose nanofibers; CNFs).

3.2 Information from Existing Literature

3.2.1 Mesothelioma and Mesothelial Cell-Related Biological Responses Caused by Asbestos

Asbestos is a well-established cause of mesothelioma following inhalation exposure. Biological responses are initiated when asbestos deposits in the lungs (Yamato 1994). Materials with low clearance by macrophage-mediated removal or low solubility in the lung are more harmful. In particular, fibers with diameters below 0.25 μm and lengths exceeding 8 μm have been shown to possess high carcinogenic potential, as described by the Stanton–Pott hypothesis (Pott et al. 1974; Stanton et al. 1977, 1981; Pott 1978). According to this hypothesis, fibrous materials beyond asbestos may exhibit carcinogenicity if they possess similar dimensions. However, not all fibrous materials meeting these criteria demonstrate carcinogenic effects in practice, indicating that fiber shape alone is insufficient and that carcinogenesis results from complex interactions with additional factors. Even among asbestos types, crocidolite (blue asbestos) and amosite (brown asbestos) exhibit carcinogenicity several tens to hundreds of times greater than that of chrysotile (white asbestos) (Nicholson and Raffn 1995; Gibbs and Berry 2008).

Following inhalation exposure, larger particles are trapped in the nasal cavity and trachea and are subsequently cleared from the body. Fibers that reach and deposit in the alveoli may migrate from the alveolar region to mesothelial tissues such as the pleura, thereby contributing to mesothelioma development. Thus, mesothelioma induction via inhalation exposure depends not only on the carcinogenic potential at the mesothelial cell level but also on deposition in the alveoli and subsequent translocation to mesothelial sites.

While the physicochemical properties of fibrous substances are critical determinants of toxicity, biological factors—including tissue-specific exposure and cell-type-specific responses—must also be considered. Cellular responses to a given substance are not uniform and vary depending on cell type. The following mechanisms have been proposed to explain asbestos-induced carcinogenesis (Toyokuni et al. 2011):

1. *Oxidative Stress Hypothesis*

   Iron present in asbestos can catalyze free radical generation, resulting in oxidative stress in the body. Crocidolite and amosite, which exhibit higher carcinogenicity, contain greater iron content and generate free radicals in the presence of hydrogen peroxide in vitro. When asbestos induces oxidative stress in vivo, increased expression of oxidative stress response proteins—such as heme oxygenase-1 (HO-1)—is observed at both cellular and tissue levels. In addition, activation of the nuclear factor erythroid 2–related factor 2 (Nrf2)–mediated pathways increases expression of antioxidant proteins (Pietrofesa et al. 2016), which mitigate oxidative stress induced by asbestos. While free radical generation by asbestos does not necessarily correlate directly with oxidative stress burden in vivo, strong or persistent free radical production that overwhelms antioxidant defenses leads to elevated reactive oxygen species (ROS) at the cellular level, oxidative damage to lipids, proteins, and nucleic acids in the body, disrupting homeostasis and ultimately leading to diseases including cancer. In rats, increased HO-1 expression in lung tissue was observed 6 months after intratracheal administration of 2 mg crocidolite (Nagatomo et al. 2005).

2. *Chromosomal Mis-segregation Hypothesis*

   Mesothelial cells possess phagocytic capability and can internalize asbestos fibers. Internalized asbestos may interfere with chromosomal segregation during cell division, leading to abnormal mitosis. However, it has been reported that macrophages and human pleural mesothelial MeT-5A cells internalize crocidolite fibers and incur DNA damage via radical production while still undergoing cell division (Jiang et al. 2008).

3. *Molecular Adsorption Hypothesis*

   Asbestos has a strong capacity to adsorb environmental substances, and it has been hypothesized that asbestos fibers act as carriers, transporting adsorbed toxic compounds into tissues or cells. According to this hypothesis, its carcinogenic potency depends partly on the nature of the adsorbed substances rather than on asbestos itself. Adsorptive properties are not unique to asbestos and are also characteristic of particulate matter—particularly industrial nanoparticles with high specific surface areas and thus higher adsorption capacity (Horie et al. 2013). Consequently, biological effects depend on the adsorbed substances rather than asbestos itself.

Collectively, these hypotheses explain the causes of asbestos toxicity, leading to inflammation, cellular damage, and eventual carcinogenesis. Among them, oxidative stress induction is considered the most critical mechanism. The pathogenicity of asbestos, including mesothelioma development, depends largely on its long-term retention in the body following exposure, resulting in sustained oxidative stress and chronic inflammation. Below is a summary of representative biomarkers associated with asbestos-induced biological responses.

Exposure of human pleural mesothelial MeT-5A cells to chrysotile at 5 $\mu g/cm^2$ for 72 h resulted in increased expression of transforming growth factor beta 1 (TGFβ1), a mediator of epithelial–mesenchymal transition (EMT) associated with fibrosis and tumor development (Turini et al. 2019). Turini et al. proposed that TGFβ1-mediated EMT may contribute to mesothelioma formation. Chrysotile exposure also induced changes in gene expression, including downregulation of cadherin-1 (CDH1). Although CDH1 abnormalities are associated with hereditary diffuse gastric cancer, their relevance to mesothelioma remains unclear.

When asbestos was administered to MeT-5A cells at 0.02 $\mu g/cm^2$ for 4 months, increased expression of matrix metalloproteinase-2 (MMP-2), a marker associated with cellular invasion, was observed (Lohcharoenkal et al. 2013). In pleural mesothelial cells exposed to crocidolite at 5 $\mu g/cm^2$ for 8 h, elevated interleukin-1 beta (IL-1β) gene expression was reported (Dragon et al. 2015).

Studies of plasma and peripheral CD4+ T cells from mesothelioma patients have reported increased levels of TGF-β, B-cell lymphoma 2 (BCL-2), and interleukin-10

(IL-10) (Maeda et al. 2008). Elevated levels of high mobility group box 1 protein (HMGB1) and tumor necrosis factor alpha (TNF-α) have also been observed in mesothelioma patients and asbestos-exposed individuals (Ying et al. 2017; Qi et al. 2013; Yang et al. 2010; Tabata et al. 2013; Napolitano et al. 2016). HMGB1 acts as a damage-associated molecular pattern protein that promotes macrophage recruitment and chronic inflammation, while TNF-α is a central inflammatory mediator, suggesting asbestos exposure increases inflammatory markers. In addition, increased serum levels of mesothelin (MSLN) (Goricar et al. 2020; Creaney et al. 2013) and osteopontin (OPN) (Pass et al. 2005) have been reported in asbestos-exposed individuals.

Although variability exists across studies, increased expression of TGFβ1, HMGB1, TNF-α, and IL-1β is consistently reported following asbestos exposure. More broadly, asbestos exposure is associated with alterations in inflammation-related, fibrosis-related, and EMT-related gene expression profiles. Increased expression of MSLN and OPN is also considered relevant to asbestos-related mesothelioma development. MSLN is currently the only mesothelioma diagnostic biomarker approved by the U.S. Food and Drug Administration (FDA), although it has low sensitivity and is approved only for monitoring tumor recurrence. At the research level, HMGB1 and OPN, in combination with MSLN, have been proposed as candidate biomarkers for asbestos-related mesothelioma (Tabata et al. 2013; Napolitano et al. 2016; Chen et al. 2017; Creaney et al. 2010).

3.2.2 *Mesothelioma and Mesothelial Cell-Related Biological Responses Induced by Exposure to Multiwalled Carbon Nanotubes*

MWCNTs exhibit substantial variability among materials, and not all MWCNTs clearly induce mesothelioma. Reports of MWCNT-induced mesothelioma are relatively limited, and many aspects of the underlying mechanisms remain unclear. Similar to asbestos, iron is considered an important contributor to MWCNT toxicity (Visalli et al. 2017). Some MWCNTs retain residual metals—such as iron, nickel, and yttrium—used as catalysts during manufacturing.

In a study where MWCNTs (Mitsui MWCNT-7; fiber length 1–20 μm, diameter 70–170 nm, containing 3500 ppm iron) were administered intraperitoneally as a single dose of 3000 μg per p53+/− knockout mouse (lacking the p53 tumor suppressor gene), mesothelioma developed in 87.5% of animals within 180 days (Takagi et al. 2008). In the same study, intraperitoneal administration of crocidolite at a comparable dose resulted in a mesothelioma incidence of 77.8% (14/18 mice). Subsequent investigations demonstrated a dose-dependent increase in mesothelioma incidence following MWCNT-7 administration in p53+/− mice (Takagi et al. 2012). Specifically, intraperitoneal doses of 300, 30, and 3 μg per p53+/− mouse resulted in mesothelioma incidence rates of 95.0% (19/20), 85.0% (17/20), and

25.0% (5/20), respectively, during a 1-year observation period. These findings indicate that certain MWCNT types possess strong mesothelioma-inducing potential. In contrast, intraperitoneal administration of four different MWCNT types to healthy mice in a contemporaneous study induced inflammatory responses and granuloma formation but did not result in mesothelioma (Poland et al. 2008).

In rat studies, intratesticular administration of MWCNT-7 resulted in peritoneal mesothelioma in 6 of 7 animals after 52 weeks (Sakamoto et al. 2009). Conversely, implantation of 10 mg of MWCNTs (fiber length 1–2 μm, diameter 10–30 nm) encapsulated in a dissolvable capsule into the rat peritoneal cavity produced granuloma formation after 12 months but did not induce mesothelioma (Varga and Szendi 2010). In another study, single intraperitoneal administration of MWCNTs (fiber length 0.7 μm, average diameter 11.3 nm, containing 19,700 ppm carbon, 4900 ppm iron, cobalt, and structural defects) to healthy rats at doses of 20 or 2 mg per animal, followed by a 2-year observation period, resulted in mesothelioma incidences of 0% (0/50) and 4.0% (2/50), respectively, with no statistically significant difference between groups (Muller et al. 2009). The authors concluded that these MWCNTs were not carcinogenic under the experimental conditions employed.

Taken together, the ability of MWCNTs to induce mesothelioma varies depending on the MWCNT type. To date, MWCNT-7—as used in the studies by Takagi et al.—has demonstrated the strongest mesothelioma induction, whereas other MWCNTs have shown weak or no such effects. A comparative intraperitoneal study in rats using MWCNTs with different diameters revealed that MWCNTs with diameters of approximately 50 nm (including MWCNT-7) induced stronger inflammatory responses and higher mesothelioma incidence than fibers with diameters around 150 nm, despite similar fiber lengths (approximately 4–6 μm) (Nagai et al. 2011). The 50-nm diameter MWCNTs were internalized by mesothelial cells and exhibited cytotoxicity, whereas the 150-nm diameter thick MWCNTs were not taken up by mesothelial cells and showed no cytotoxic effects. Furthermore, tangled MWCNTs (fiber length 3 μm, diameter 2–20 nm) were less readily internalized and did not induce mesothelioma (Nagai et al. 2011, 2013). Similarly, a study administering MWCNTs of different shapes intraperitoneally to rats revealed that straight MWCNTs induced mesothelioma at earlier stages and with higher frequency than curved MWCNTs, which showed delayed mesothelioma development (Rittinghausen et al. 2014). Collectively, these findings suggest that mesothelial cell responsiveness to MWCNTs—particularly phagocytic uptake—is a critical determinant of MWCNT-induced mesothelioma, and that MWCNT fiber diameter, rigidity, and agglomeration state play important roles. In addition, host-related biological factors, such as the presence or absence of tumor suppressor gene abnormalities, may influence susceptibility to mesothelioma induction by MWCNTs. It is necessary to design experimental models based on the exposure scenarios considered. While many studies have focused on histological evaluations with carcinogenesis as the endpoint, the molecular inflammatory processes leading to mesothelioma remain incompletely understood.

Below is a summary of candidate biomarkers identified from epidemiological studies and animal experiments. Blood analyses of workers exposed to MWCNTs have reported increased levels of TGFβ1, TNF-α, and IL-1β, similar to patterns observed following asbestos exposure; however, no mesothelioma cases have been reported in these populations and the clinical relevance of these findings remains uncertain (Shvedova et al. 2016; Fatkhutdinova et al. 2016). Long-term exposure of human pleural mesothelial MeT-5A cells to MWCNTs (0.02 $\mu g/cm^2$ for 4 months) resulted in increased MMP-2 expression, comparable to responses observed following asbestos exposure (Lohcharoenkal et al. 2013). In a rat study where MWCNT-7—previously reported to induce mesothelioma following intratracheal administration—was administered intratracheally at 0.5 mg per rat and the animals were observed for 2 years, increased levels of the inflammatory markers CC chemokine ligand 2 (CCL2) and CC chemokine ligand 3 (CCL3) was detected in lung tissue, along with significant increases in HMGB1 in pleural lavage fluid (Saleh et al. 2022). In this experiment, many animals died prior to the 2-year endpoint due to mesothelioma; however, those surviving to 2 years did not develop mesothelioma. In rats with mesothelioma observed 52 weeks after MWCNT-7 administration, increased MSLN expression was also detected, suggesting a correlation (Sakamoto et al. 2010). Although the available dataset is smaller than that for asbestos, highly toxic MWCNTs capable of inducing mesothelioma exhibit gene expression responses overlapping with those observed for asbestos exposure, including inflammatory markers and mesothelioma-associated biomarkers such as MSLN and HMGB1.

Figure 3.1 summarizes candidate biomarkers associated with asbestos and MWCNT exposure based on previous reports.

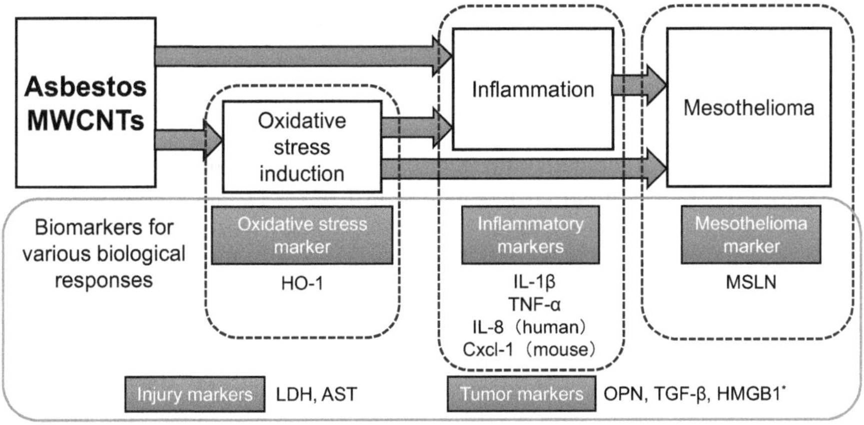

Fig. 3.1 Candidate biomarkers for asbestos and MWCNT exposure based on the existing literature
*HMGB1 is reported to increase not only due to mesothelioma development but also as an inflammatory mediator

3.3 Key Findings from the NEDO Project

To date, no studies have verified mesothelioma development induced by CNFs. Accordingly, within the NEDO project (FY2020–2024), the mesothelioma induction potential of CNFs was evaluated via a 2-year in vivo intraperitoneal administration study in mice and in vitro mesothelial cell assays (Horie et al. 2025). Three CNF types were examined: mechanically fibrillated CNFs, TEMPO-oxidized CNFs, and phosphorylated CNFs.

The dispersion state of fibrous materials such as CNFs is a critical factor in safety assessment. Agglomeration or aggregation of fibers, as well as fiber breakage resulting from excessive ultrasonication, can lead to misinterpretation of inherent biological effects (Zhang et al. 2024). In addition, microbial contamination must also be considered when handling CNFs. In this study, samples were irradiated with gamma rays at absorbed doses selected to avoid sterilization while preserving the physical properties of CNFs (Horie et al. 2023; Ogura et al. 2025). The physicochemical properties of the CNF dispersions used for administration were also characterized to confirm the specific features of each CNF type.

3.3.1 Intraperitoneal Administration Test in Mice

B6C3F1 mice, which are commonly used in carcinogenicity studies and have an approximate 2-year survival rate of 70% (Yafune et al. 2010), were used in this study. Dispersions of the three CNF types were administered intraperitoneally to 6-week-old B6C3F1 mice at doses of 0.1 and 1.0 mg, followed by observation for up to 2 years (Horie et al. 2025). Because inflammation induction is considered a critical factor in mesothelioma development by asbestos and certain MWCNTs, necropsies were conducted at 1 month, 3 months, 6 months, and 1 year postadministration. Evaluations focused on inflammatory responses and carcinogenic markers, including mesothelioma-associated biomarkers. Given the intraperitoneal exposure route, aspartate aminotransferase (AST) was measured as a liver injury marker; IL-1β, C-X-C motif chemokine ligand 1 (Cxcl-1), and TNF-α were measured as inflammatory markers; MSLN was evaluated as a mesothelioma-associated marker; and HMGB1, OPN, and TGF-β were assessed as tumor-related markers. Cxcl-1 is functionally similar to human interleukin-8 (IL-8). HMGB1 has been reported to promote pleural mesothelioma progression (Wang et al. 2019; Suarez et al. 2023). Blood HMGB1 concentrations were measured at 6 months, 1 year, and 2 years. At necropsy, blood and intraperitoneal lavage fluid were collected by washing the peritoneal cavity with 5 mL of phosphate-buffered saline. The digestive organs, including the liver and kidneys, were excised, fixed in 10% formalin, and subjected to hematoxylin and eosin staining for histopathological examination.

The biomarker results are summarized in Table 3.1. Throughout the entire observation period, no statistically significant differences were observed in AST or

Table 3.1 Summary of results for each biomarker after intraperitoneal administration of CNFs

Biomarker category	Biomarker	Mechanical fibrillated CNFs	TEMPO-oxidized CNFs	Phosphorylated CNFs
Liver Injury Marker	AST	No significant difference	No significant difference	No significant difference
Inflammation Marker	IL-1β	No significant difference	No significant difference	No significant difference
Inflammation Marker	Cxcl-1	No significant difference	No significant difference	No significant difference
Inflammation Marker	TNF-α	No significant difference	No significant difference	No significant difference
Mesothelioma Marker	MSLN	No significant increase (decreased after 1 year)	No significant increase (decreased after 1 year)	No significant increase (decreased after 1 year)
Tumor Marker	HMGB1	No significant difference	Significant increase after 1 year; no difference at 6 months and 2 years	Significant increase in low-dose group after 2 years ($p < 0.05$)
Tumor Marker	OPN	No significant difference	No significant difference	Significant increase in high-dose group after 3 months ($p < 0.01$); no increase at other time points
Tumor Marker	TGF-β	No significant difference	No significant difference	No significant difference
Histopathological Observation	Mesothelioma Occurrence	Not observed	Not observed	Not observed
Histopathological Observation	Inflammation and Other Findings	No inflammation. CNF adhesion to liver and spleen throughout the study period.	None	None

The results are presented in comparison with the untreated control group. HMGB1 was measured from 6 months onward and TGF-β was measured at 2 years. Based on the results of Horie et al. (2025)

inflammatory marker levels in any CNF-treated group at either dose compared with controls. OPN levels showed no significant differences from controls throughout the tested period in mice administered mechanically fibrillated or TEMPO-oxidized CNFs. In contrast, phosphorylated CNFs induced a significant increase in OPN at 3 months in the high-dose group; however, no significant differences were observed at 6 months or at later time points up to 2 years. MSLN tended to decrease in the CNF-treated groups compared with controls at 1 year, and no significant increases were observed at any time point. Mice administered TEMPO-oxidized CNFs exhibited a significant increase in blood HMGB1 levels at 1 year, but this difference was not maintained at 2 years. In the phosphorylated CNF groups, a significant increase in HMGB1 was observed at 2 years in the low-dose group. No significant differences in HMGB1 levels were observed in mice administered mechanically fibrillated CNFs. Blood TGF-β concentrations at 2 years also showed no significant differences compared with controls.

Overall, no significant changes were observed in inflammatory markers. Although transient fluctuations were noted in certain tumor-related biomarkers, mesothelioma was not observed in any organ—including the peritoneum—throughout the 2-year study period in any CNF-treated group. Moreover, no marked inflammation or other pathological findings attributable to CNF administration were observed at any time point.

Notably, in mice administered mechanically fibrillated CNFs, white deposits were observed on the liver and spleen in the high-dose group. These deposits were present from 1 month through 2 years postadministration. Enzymatic evaluation using cellulase suggested that the deposits consisted of cellulose. These findings indicate that mechanically fibrillated CNFs administered intraperitoneally remained in the peritoneal cavity for the 2-year duration. Even in animals exhibiting these deposits, no increases in inflammatory or tumor-related biomarkers were detected, nor were any notable pathological changes observed.

3.3.2 Cell Culture Tests

CNF dispersions were administered to MeT-5A cells, a human-derived mesothelial cell line, and to THP-1 cells differentiated into macrophages to evaluate the cellular responses (Horie et al. 2025). Cell viability was evaluated via the WST-1 assay, and cytotoxicity was assessed by measuring cell membrane damage via the lactate dehydrogenase (LDH) assay. In addition, the potential for inflammation induction—a key event in mesothelioma development—was evaluated by measuring cytokine production.

The results of these cell culture tests are summarized in Table 3.2. None of the CNF dispersions exhibited cytotoxicity toward either MeT-5A or THP-1 cells. In MeT-5A cells, no induction of inflammatory cytokines such as IL-1β and TNF-α, nor of the neutrophil chemokine IL-8, was observed, indicating minimal responsiveness of mesothelial cells to CNF exposure. In contrast, THP-1 cells exhibited induction of IL-8 following treatment with 100 μg/mL CNF dispersions, with the strongest response observed for mechanically fibrillated CNFs. Induction of IL-1β was also detected in THP-1 cells. However, the oxidative stress marker HO-1 was not significantly induced by CNF treatment in either cell type. Furthermore, comprehensive gene expression analysis using next-generation sequencing of CNF-treated cells revealed no upregulation of inflammation-related genes or other significant changes in gene expression profiles. Taken together, these results indicate low responsiveness of mesothelial cells to CNF dispersions, with no marked biological effects, whereas macrophages exhibited cytokine induction, suggesting a

Table 3.2 Summary of cell culture test results following CNF exposure

Targeted cellular effects	Biomarker	Mechanical fibrillated CNFs	TEMPO-oxidized CNFs	Phosphorylated CNFs
Cytotoxicity	Cell Viability	No significant difference	No significant difference	No significant difference
	Cell Membrane Damage	No significant difference	No significant difference	No significant difference
Oxidative stress induction	HO-1	No significant difference	No significant difference	No significant difference
Proinflammatory response	IL-8	Slight decrease	Slight decrease	Slight decrease
	IL-1β	Not detected	Not detected	Not detected

Each CNF sample was administered to the cells at concentrations of 10 or 100 μg/mL and incubated for 24 h. Based on the results of Horie et al. (2025)

potential inflammatory effect of CNF dispersions. Importantly, in the corresponding in vivo studies with a 2-year observation period, no inflammation was observed even at high doses, and no evidence of sustained inflammation was detected. Although CNFs were capable of inducing inflammatory cytokines and chemokines in macrophages under in vitro conditions, these findings suggest that CNF exposure is unlikely to cause persistent and significant inflammatory responses leading to carcinogenesis, including mesothelioma.

3.4 Summary

Asbestos and certain types of MWCNTs are well-established inducers of mesothelioma. Proposed mechanisms underlying asbestos-induced mesothelioma include oxidative stress induction, disruption of cell division, and adsorption of harmful substances from the environment. Phagocytosis by mesothelial cells and long-term retention of these substances in the body without effective clearance are also considered critical factors in mesothelioma development. Regarding MWCNTs, fibers with diameters of approximately 50 nm are readily internalized by mesothelial cells and induce mesothelioma with high probability, whereas fibers with diameters of approximately 150 nm or tangled forms are not efficiently internalized and do not induce mesothelioma. These findings highlight the importance of fiber shape, rigidity, and agglomeration state. In addition, iron contamination has been identified as an important contributor to mesothelioma induction by both asbestos and MWCNTs, as retained iron can promote persistent oxidative stress, chronic inflammation, and subsequent carcinogenesis. Candidate biomarkers for monitoring biological effects leading to mesothelioma development include HMGB1, MSLN, OPN, TGFβ1, TNF-α, and IL-1β.

For CNFs, no studies have previously verified mesothelioma development. Accordingly, the NEDO project (FY2020–2024) evaluated their mesothelioma induction potential using long-term intraperitoneal administration studies in mice, as well as cultured cell assays involving mesothelial cells and macrophages. Three CNF types—mechanically fibrillated CNFs, TEMPO-oxidized CNFs, and phosphorylated CNFs—were administered intraperitoneally to mice and observed for 2 years. No mesothelioma was detected in any of the CNF-treated groups. Although induction of chemokines and inflammatory cytokines was observed in macrophages under in vitro conditions, no inflammation was observed in the in vivo studies from 1 month postadministration onward. Inflammatory markers and mesothelioma-related biomarkers reported to increase in blood following asbestos exposure did not show any elevation throughout the observation period, and no notable pathological findings attributable to CNF administration were observed. Collectively, these results indicate that, for the three CNF types tested, no sustained inflammation—a key initiating event for mesothelioma—was induced, and no mesothelioma development occurred under the conditions evaluated.

References

Chen Z, Gaudino G, Pass HI, Carbone M, Yang H (2017) Diagnostic and prognostic biomarkers for malignant mesothelioma: an update. Transl Lung Cancer Res 6(3):259–269. https://doi.org/10.21037/tlcr.2017.05.06

Chen Z, Cai Y, Ou T, Zhou H, Li H, Wang Z, Cai K (2024) Global burden of mesothelioma attributable to occupational asbestos exposure in 204 countries and territories: 1990–2019. J Cancer Res Clin Oncol 150:282. https://doi.org/10.1007/s00432-024-05802-6

Creaney J, Olsen NJ, Brims F, Dick IM, Musk AW, de Klerk NH, Skates SJ, Robinson BWS (2010) Serum mesothelin for early detection of asbestos-induced cancer malignant mesothelioma. Cancer Epidemiol Biomarkers Prev 19(9):2238–2246. https://doi.org/10.1158/1055-9965.EPI-10-0346

Creaney J, Sneddon S, Dick IM, Dare H, Boudville N, Musk AW, Skates SJ, Robinson BWS (2013) Comparison of the diagnostic accuracy of the MSLN gene products, mesothelin and megakaryocyte potentiating factor, as biomarkers for mesothelioma in pleural effusions and serum. Dis Markers 35(2):119–127. https://doi.org/10.1155/2013/874212

Dragon J, Thompson J, MacPherson M, Shukla A (2015) Differential susceptibility of human pleural and peritoneal mesothelial cells to asbestos exposure. J Cell Biochem 116(8):1540–1552. https://doi.org/10.1002/jcb.25095

Fatkhutdinova LM, Khaliullin TO, Vasil'yeva OL, Zalyalov RR, Mustafin IG, Kisin ER, Birch ME, Yanamala N, Shvedova AA (2016) Fibrosis biomarkers in workers exposed to MWCNTs. Toxicol Appl Pharmacol 299:125–131. https://doi.org/10.1016/j.taap.2016.02.016

Gibbs GW, Berry G (2008) Mesothelioma and asbestos. Regul Toxicol Pharmacol 52(1_Suppl):S223–S231. https://doi.org/10.1016/j.yrtph.2007.10.003

Goricar K, Kovac V, Dodic-Fikfak M, Dolzan V, Franko A (2020) Evaluation of soluble mesothelin-related peptides and MSLN genetic variability in asbestos-related diseases. Radiol Oncol 54(1):86–95. https://doi.org/10.2478/raon-2020-0011

Horie M, Kato H, Iwahashi H (2013) Cellular effects of manufactured nanoparticles: effect of adsorption ability of nanoparticles. Arch Toxicol 87(5):771–781. https://doi.org/10.1007/s00204-013-1033-5

Horie M, Fujita K, Endoh S, Sugino S, Maru J, Moriyama A, Ogura I (2023) Contaminant microorganisms in the *in vitro* evaluation of cellular responses of cellulose nanofibers and their microbial inactivation using gamma irradiation. Toxicol Mech Methods 33(9):741–754. https://doi.org/10.1080/15376516.2023.2238061

Horie M, Sugino S, Fujita K, Endoh S, Maru J, Matsuzawa T, Ogura I (2025) Evaluation of inflammatory and mesothelioma-related responses in mice following the intraperitoneal administration of cellulose nanofibers. NanoImpact 38:100561. https://doi.org/10.1016/j.impact.2025.100561
Inai K, Takeshima Y, Kushitani K (2007) Pathology of mesothelioma. Jpn J Lung Cancer 47(3):223–232. (in Japanese)
Jiang L, Nagai H, Ohara H, Hara S, Tachibana M, Hirano S, Shinohara Y, Kohyama N, Akatsuka S, Toyokuni S (2008) Characteristics and modifying factors of asbestos-induced oxidative DNA damage. Cancer Sci 99(11):2142–2151. https://doi.org/10.1111/j.1349-7006.2008.00934.x
Lohcharoenkal W, Wang L, Stueckle TA, Dinu CZ, Castranova V, Liu Y, Rojanasakul Y (2013) Chronic exposure to carbon nanotubes induces invasion of human mesothelial cells through matrix metalloproteinase-2. ACS Nano 7(9):7711–7723. https://doi.org/10.1021/nn402241b
Maeda M, Miura Y, Nishimura Y, Murakami S, Hayashi H, Kumagai N, Hatayama T, Katoh M, Miyahara N, Yamamoto S, Fukuoka K, Kishimoto T, Nakano T, Otsuki T (2008) Immunological changes in mesothelioma patients and their experimental detection. Clin Med Circ Respirat Pulm Med 2:11–17. https://doi.org/10.4137/CCRPM.S577
Muller J, Delos M, Panin N, Rabolli V, Huaux F, Lison D (2009) Absence of carcinogenic response to multiwall carbon nanotubes in a 2-year bioassay in the peritoneal cavity of the rat. Toxicol Sci 110(2):442–448. https://doi.org/10.1093/toxsci/kfp100
Nagai H, Okazaki Y, Chew SH, Misawa N, Yamashita Y, Akatsuka S, Ishihara T, Yamashita K, Yoshikawa Y, Yasui H, Jiang L, Ohara H, Takahashi T, Ichihara G, Kostarelos K, Miyata Y, Shinohara H, Toyokuni S (2011) Diameter and rigidity of multiwalled carbon nanotubes are critical factors in mesothelial injury and carcinogenesis. Proc Natl Acad Sci USA 108(49):E1330–E1338. https://doi.org/10.1073/pnas.1110013108
Nagai H, Okazaki Y, Chew SH, Misawa N, Miyata Y, Shinohara H, Toyokuni S (2013) Intraperitoneal administration of tangled multiwalled carbon nanotubes of 15 nm in diameter does not induce mesothelial carcinogenesis in rats. Pathol Int 63(9):457–462. https://doi.org/10.1111/pin.12093
Nagatomo H, Morimoto Y, Oyabu T, Hirohashi M, Ogami A, Yamato H, Kuroda K, Higashi T, Tanaka I (2005) Expression of heme oxygenase-1 in the lungs of rats exposed to crocidolite asbestos. Inhal Toxicol 17(6):293–296. https://doi.org/10.1080/08958370590922580
Napolitano A, Antoine DJ, Pellegrini L, Baumann F, Pagano I, Pastorino S, Goparaju CM, Prokrym K, Canino C, Pass HI, Carbone M, Yang H (2016) HMGB1 and its hyperacetylated isoform are sensitive and specific serum biomarkers to detect asbestos exposure and to identify mesothelioma patients. Clin Cancer Res 22(12):3087–3096. https://doi.org/10.1158/1078-0432.CCR-15-1130
Nicholson WJ, Raffn E (1995) Recent data on cancer due to asbestos in the U.S.A. and Denmark. Med Lav 86(5):393–410
Ogura I, Moriyama A, Iizumi Y, Endoh S, Fujita K, Horie M, Okazaki T, Matsuzawa T (2025) Effect of gamma irradiation on cellulose nanofibers. J Wood Sci 71(1):37. https://doi.org/10.1186/s10086-025-02215-y
Pass HI, Lott D, Lonardo F, Harbut M, Liu Z, Tang N, Carbone M, Webb C, Wali A (2005) Asbestos exposure, pleural mesothelioma, and serum osteopontin levels. N Engl J Med 353(15):1564–1573. https://doi.org/10.1056/NEJMoa051185
Pietrofesa RA, Velalopoulou A, Albelda SM, Christofidou-Solomidou M (2016) Asbestos induces oxidative stress and activation of Nrf2 signaling in murine macrophages: Chemopreventive role of the synthetic lignan secoisolariciresinol diglucoside (LGM2605). Int J Mol Sci 17(3):322. https://doi.org/10.3390/ijms17030322
Poland CA, Duffin R, Kinloch I, Maynard A, Wallace WAH, Seaton A, Stone V, Brown S, Macnee W, Donaldson K (2008) Carbon nanotubes introduced into the abdominal cavity of mice show asbestos-like pathogenicity in a pilot study. Nat Nanotechnol 3(7):423–428. https://doi.org/10.1038/nnano.2008.111
Pott F (1978) Some aspects on the dosimetry of the carcinogenic potency of asbestos and other fibrous dusts. Staub-Reinh Luft 38:486–490

Pott F, Huth F, Friedrichs KH (1974) Tumorigenic effect of fibrous dusts in experimental animals. Environ Health Perspect 9:313–315. https://doi.org/10.1289/ehp.749313

Qi F, Okimoto G, Jube S, Napolitano A, Pass HI, Laczko R, Demay RM, Khan G, Tiirikainen M, Rinaudo C, Croce A, Yang H, Gaudino G, Carbone M (2013) Continuous exposure to chrysotile asbestos can cause transformation of human mesothelial cells via HMGB1 and TNF-α signaling. Am J Pathol 183(5):1654–1666. https://doi.org/10.1016/j.ajpath.2013.07.029

Rittinghausen S, Hackbarth A, Creutzenberg O, Ernst H, Heinrich U, Leonhardt A, Schaudien D (2014) The carcinogenic effect of various multi-walled carbon nanotubes (MWCNTs) after intraperitoneal injection in rats. Part Fibre Toxicol 11:59. https://doi.org/10.1186/s12989-014-0059-z

Sakamoto Y, Nakae D, Fukumori N, Tayama K, Maekawa A, Imai K, Hirose A, Nishimura T, Ohashi N, Ogata A (2009) Induction of mesothelioma by a single intrascrotal administration of multi-wall carbon nanotube in intact male Fischer 344 rats. J Toxicol Sci 34(1):65–76. https://doi.org/10.2131/jts.34.65

Sakamoto Y, Dai N, Hagiwara Y, Satoh K, Ohashi N, Fukamachi K, Tsuda H, Hirose A, Nishimura T, Hino O, Ogata A (2010) Serum level of expressed in renal carcinoma (ERC)/mesothelin in rats with mesothelial proliferative lesions induced by multi-wall carbon nanotube (MWCNT). J Toxicol Sci 35(2):265–270. https://doi.org/10.2131/jts.35.265

Saleh DM, Luo S, Ahmed OHM, Alexander DB, Alexander WT, Gunasekaran S, El-Gazzar AM, Abdelgied M, Numano T, Takase H, Ohnishi M, Tomono S, Hady RHAE, Fukamachi K, Kanno J, Hirose A, Xu J, Suzuki S, Naiki-Ito A, Takahashi S, Tsuda H (2022) Assessment of the toxicity and carcinogenicity of double-walled carbon nanotubes in the rat lung after intratracheal instillation: a two-year study. Part Fibre Toxicol 19(1):30. https://doi.org/10.1186/s12989-022-00469-8

Shvedova AA, Yanamala N, Kisin ER, Khailullin TO, Birch ME, Fatkhutdinova LM (2016) Integrated analysis of dysregulated ncRNA and mRNA expression profiles in humans exposed to carbon nanotubes. PLoS One 11(3):e0150628. https://doi.org/10.1371/journal.pone.0150628

Stanton MF, Laynard M, Tegeris A, Miller E, May M, Kent E (1977) Carcinogenicity of fibrous glass: pleural response in the rat in relation to fiber dimension. J Natl Cancer Inst 58(3):587–603. https://doi.org/10.1093/jnci/58.3.587

Stanton MF, Layard M, Tegeris A, Miller E, May M, Morgan E, Smith A (1981) Relation of particle dimension to carcinogenicity in amphibole asbestoses and other fibrous minerals. J Natl Cancer Inst 67(5):965–975

Suarez JS, Novelli F, Goto K, Ehara M, Steele M, Kim JH, Zolondick AA, Xue J, Xu R, Saito M, Pastorino S, Minaai M, Takanishi Y, Emi M, Pagano I, Wakeham A, Berger T, Pass HI, Gaudino G, Mak TW, Carbone M, Yang H (2023) HMGB1 released by mesothelial cells drives the development of asbestos-induced mesothelioma. Proc Natl Acad Sci USA 120(39):e2307999120. https://doi.org/10.1073/pnas.2307999120

Tabata C, Shibata E, Tabata R, Kanemura S, Mikami K, Nogi Y, Masachika E, Nishizaki T, Nakano T (2013) Serum HMGB1 as a prognostic marker for malignant pleural mesothelioma. BMC Cancer 13:205. https://doi.org/10.1186/1471-2407-13-205

Takagi A, Hirose A, Nishimura T, Fukumori N, Ogata A, Ohashi N, Kitajima S, Kanno J (2008) Induction of mesothelioma in p53+/− mouse by intraperitoneal application of multi-wall carbon nanotube. J Toxicol Sci 33(1):105–116. https://doi.org/10.2131/jts.33.105

Takagi A, Hirose A, Futakuchi M, Tsuda H, Kanno J (2012) Dose-dependent mesothelioma induction by intraperitoneal administration of multi-wall carbon nanotubes in p53 heterozygous mice. Cancer Sci 103(8):1440–1444. https://doi.org/10.1111/j.1349-7006.2012.02318.x

Toyokuni S, Jiang L, Hu Q, Nagai H, Okazaki Y, Akatsuka S, Yamashita Y (2011) Mechanisms of asbestos-induced carcinogenesis. Nihon Eiseigaku Zasshi 66(3):562–567. https://doi.org/10.1265/jjh.66.562. (in Japanese)

Turini S, Bergandi L, Gazzano E, Prato M, Aldieri E (2019) Epithelial to mesenchymal transition in human mesothelial cells exposed to asbestos fibers: role of TGF-β as mediator of malignant mesothelioma development or metastasis via EMT event. Int J Mol Sci 20(1):150. https://doi.org/10.3390/ijms20010150

Varga C, Szendi K (2010) Carbon nanotubes induce granulomas but not mesotheliomas. In Vivo 24(2):153–156

Visalli G, Facciolà A, Iannazzo D, Piperno A, Pistone A, Di Pietro A (2017) The role of the iron catalyst in the toxicity of multi-walled carbon nanotubes (MWCNTs). J Trace Elem Med Biol 43:153–160. https://doi.org/10.1016/j.jtemb.2017.01.005

Wang Y, Jiang Z, Yan J, Ying S (2019) HMGB1 as a potential biomarker and therapeutic target for malignant mesothelioma. Dis Markers 2019:4183157. https://doi.org/10.1155/2019/4183157

Yafune A, Kuroiwa Y, Yamamoto S, Nakamura N, Oshima Y, Masubuchi Y, Okazaki S (2010) Comparison of background data between ICR and B6C3F1 mice in carcinogenicity studies. In: The 37th annual meeting of the Japanese Society of Toxicology, p 110. https://doi.org/10.14869/toxp.37.0.310.0. (in Japanese)

Yamato H (1994) Biological effects of inhaled fibrous particles. Earozoru Kenkyu 9(3):215–220. (in Japanese)

Yang H, Rivera Z, Jube S, Nasu M, Bertino P, Goparaju C, Franzoso G, Lotze MT, Krausz T, Pass HI, Bianchi ME, Carbone M (2010) Programmed necrosis induced by asbestos in human mesothelial cells causes high-mobility group box 1 protein release and resultant inflammation. Proc Natl Acad Sci USA 107(28):12611–12616. https://doi.org/10.1073/pnas.1006542107

Ying S, Jiang Z, He X, Yu M, Chen R, Chen J, Ru G, Chen Y, Chen W, Zhu L, Li T, Zhang Y, Guo X, Yin X, Zhang X, Lou J (2017) Serum HMGB1 as a potential biomarker for patients with asbestos-related diseases. Dis Markers 2017:5756102. https://doi.org/10.1155/2017/5756102

Zhang Y, Fox DM, Ong KJ, Ede J, Sayes C, Kangas H, Ilona L, Goergen M, Moon R, Shatkin JA (2024) Limitations of recent cellulose studies: how overzealous dispersion technique, fluorescence labeling and interpretation limit the findings of recent safety assessments for cellulose materials. Trends Food Sci Technol 151:104620. https://doi.org/10.1016/j.tifs.2024.104620

Chapter 4
Inhalation Effects: Pulmonary Responses and Long-Term Considerations

Katsuhide Fujita and Akihiro Moriyama

Abstract Inhalation exposure is a primary route of concern for nanocellulose materials (NCMs), including cellulose nanofibrils (CNFs, also referred to as cellulose nanofibers) and cellulose nanocrystals (CNCs), owing to their respirable size and expanding industrial and consumer use. This chapter provides an integrated assessment of pulmonary responses and long-term considerations associated with NCM inhalation, synthesizing evidence from the published literature with findings from studies commissioned by the New Energy and Industrial Technology Development Organization (NEDO). Studies on cellulose and microcrystalline cellulose provide a toxicological context suggesting that fibrous cellulose may induce transient pulmonary inflammation following intratracheal instillation. Across animal and in vitro studies, CNFs generally elicit milder pulmonary inflammation than CNCs and substantially weaker responses than rigid fibrous nanomaterials such as multi-walled carbon nanotubes (MWCNTs), as well as other hazardous fibrous materials including asbestos. Reported effects include acute neutrophilic inflammation, cytokine modulation, and oxidative stress–related responses. Overall, current evidence indicates a comparatively low inhalation hazard for NCMs, while highlighting remaining uncertainties related to biopersistence, chronic low-dose exposure, and material-specific properties influencing long-term toxicity.

Keywords Nanocellulose materials (NCMs) · Cellulose nanofibrils (CNFs) · Inhalation exposure · Inhalation toxicity · Pulmonary inflammation · Intratracheal instillation · Pulmonary retention

K. Fujita (✉) · A. Moriyama
Research Institute of Science for Safety and Sustainability (RISS), National Institute of Advanced Industrial Science and Technology (AIST), Tsukuba, Ibaraki, Japan
e-mail: ka-fujita@aist.go.jp; moriyama-akihiro@aist.go.jp

I. Ogura, K. Fujita (eds.), *Nanocellulose Materials*,
https://doi.org/10.1007/978-981-92-2148-6_4

4.1 Introduction

Ensuring the safe use of nanocellulose materials (NCMs)—including cellulose nanofibrils (CNFs; also referred to as cellulose nanofibers) and cellulose nanocrystals (CNCs)—is essential for their practical application and societal implementation. Potential exposure may occur not only during manufacturing and processing, but also through consumer products, such as sprays, and across diverse application areas including housing, packaging, and agriculture. Among the possible exposure routes, respiratory exposure is of particular concern, making the design and evaluation of inhalation toxicity studies a critical component of safety assurance.

Understanding the inhalation effects of NCMs is essential for protecting occupational health and for establishing a scientific basis for minimizing potential risks to consumers and the environment. Accordingly, this chapter first reviews the existing literature on the inhalation effects of cellulose and microcrystalline cellulose (MCC), providing foundational insight into their biological impacts. It then summarizes current research trends related to NCM inhalation effects, with particular attention to nanoscale-specific toxicities and proposed mechanisms of action. In addition, findings from animal studies and in vitro assays conducted within the New Energy and Industrial Technology Development Organization (NEDO) projects are presented to clarify the current status and remaining challenges in the evaluation of NCM inhalation effects. Special emphasis is placed on the relationships between NCM physicochemical properties and pulmonary responses, together with mechanistic considerations underlying toxicity expression. Finally, the chapter synthesizes these findings and discusses future research needs and challenges.

For the evaluation of chemical inhalation toxicity, the Organisation for Economic Co-operation and Development (OECD) test guidelines (TGs) provide standardized methods for inhalation toxicity testing, including:

- TG 403: Acute inhalation toxicity (OECD 2024)
- TG 412: 28-day subacute inhalation toxicity (OECD 2018a)
- TG 413: 90-day subchronic inhalation toxicity (OECD 2018b)

These tests involve aerosolizing the test substance and exposing animals via whole-body or nose-only inhalation. However, for insoluble nanomaterials such as NCMs, stable aerosol generation over extended periods and precise control of exposure concentrations present significant technical challenges, requiring specialized equipment and expertise. Consequently, the costs and time requirements associated with these studies are substantial, and the number of institutions capable of conducting them remains limited.

To date, no OECD TG-compliant whole-body inhalation exposure studies of CNFs have been reported, although some examples exist for CNCs. As alternatives, simpler inhalation exposure methods—such as oropharyngeal aspiration (administration of a suspension into the pharynx to reach the lungs by aspiration) and intratracheal instillation (direct administration of a suspension into the trachea)—have been employed in numerous NCM studies (see Sects. 4.2.2 and 4.3.3 for more details). Furthermore, under the NEDO project (FY2020–2024), a nose-only inhalation exposure study was conducted in rats at the University of Fukui, with the results discussed in Sect. 4.3.4.

In vitro cell-based assays offer a complementary approach, enabling shorter study durations and lower costs compared with animal experiments and thus improving accessibility for smaller research facilities. Although reports on NCM cytotoxicity and pulmonary-related in vitro assays remain limited, such methods are increasingly recognized as rapid and practical screening tools for inhalation hazard assessment. The development and validation of these approaches have also been actively pursued within the NEDO projects (see Sects. 4.2.3 and 4.3.3).

4.2 Information from Existing Literature

4.2.1 Evaluation of Pulmonary Responses of Cellulose and MCC

Cellulose and MCC have generally been regarded as biologically inert materials. However, experimental studies have shown that intratracheal instillation may induce pulmonary inflammation, fibrosis, and granuloma formation. Although such inflammatory responses may be transient, repeated or high-dose exposures can result in chronic effects, underscoring the importance of comprehensive toxicological assessment using both animal models and cultured cell assays.

Tátrai et al. (1995) reported that exposure to pine wood dust and cellulose induced granulomatous inflammation and fibrosis, whereas wood dust extracts lacking fibrous components did not elicit such effects, suggesting that cellulose fibers may contribute to pulmonary fibrotic responses. Cellulose exposure also stimulated hydrogen peroxide and superoxide anion production in leukocytes, suggesting a fibrosis-promoting mechanism mediated by oxidative stress.

Tátrai et al. (1996) demonstrated that a single intratracheal instillation of cellulose (15 mg/rat) caused granulomatous alveolitis and increased immunoglobulin A (IgA) levels in bronchoalveolar lavage fluid (BALF). Histopathological findings included damage to type I alveolar epithelial cells and incomplete repair of type II cells, indicating disruption of the alveolar–capillary barrier and tissue responses associated with fibrotic remodeling.

Adamis et al. (1997) observed early interstitial edema and inflammation following intratracheal instillation, which progressed to fibrotic pneumonia after 1 month. In contrast, in vitro assays using the same material showed no clear macrophage toxicity, highlighting discrepancies between in vivo and in vitro responses.

Nagato et al. (2008) evaluated pulmonary responses to intratracheally administered MCC in BALB/c mice over a 30-day period. MCC induced an acute, neutrophil-dominated inflammatory response with transient alveolar collapse, edema, and impaired lung mechanics. These effects resolved by day 30 despite particle persistence, indicating that the pulmonary response was largely self-limiting and reversible.

Milton et al. (1990) compared lung toxicity induced by cotton dust, cellulose, and endotoxin in hamsters. Endotoxin caused emphysema-like changes, whereas cellulose induced reduced lung elasticity, granuloma formation, and septal thickening. Cotton dust produced combined effects of both cellulose and endotoxin. These findings suggest that although cellulose is generally considered biologically inert, it can induce pulmonary inflammatory and fibrotic responses under certain exposure conditions.

4.2.2 Pulmonary Responses to CNFs and CNCs: Evidence from Animal Studies

Recent reviews highlight that NCMs, including CNFs and CNCs, generally exhibit lower pulmonary toxicity compared with MWCNTs or asbestos. Nevertheless, important knowledge gaps remain regarding biopersistence, clearance kinetics, and long-term effects.

Ede et al. (2019) reported that short-term inhalation exposure to CNFs induced transient inflammatory responses resembling those induced by conventional cellulose and other poorly soluble, low-toxicity dusts; however, these responses were markedly less severe than those induced by MWCNTs or asbestos.

Ventura et al. (2020) revealed that CNFs and CNCs generally exhibit low cellular uptake and have not been conclusively shown to induce oxidative stress, pronounced cytotoxicity, or genotoxicity. Long CNF fibers tend to be less readily phagocytosed by macrophages, suggesting low inflammation-inducing potential.

Conversely, some studies have reported CNF-induced DNA damage in vitro and chromosomal abnormalities in vivo, indicating possible genotoxic effects under certain conditions. CNCs, which are typically rod-shaped, have been associated with moderate to severe inflammatory responses, particularly when surface chemistry modifications influence macrophage interactions. Overall, CNFs tend to induce milder inflammatory responses than CNCs.

Rodent studies consistently demonstrate that carbon nanotubes (CNTs) cause more severe pulmonary outcomes—including interstitial fibrosis, granuloma formation, bronchoalveolar hyperplasia, and carcinogenicity—than CNFs or CNCs. These differences are attributed to variations in rigidity, aspect ratio, and surface properties.

Since 2017, various studies have employed diverse animal species, exposure routes, and durations, including (see Table 4.1 for details):

- 28-day oropharyngeal aspiration tests in mice (Ilves et al. 2018)
- 24-h and 14-day aspiration studies (Catalán et al. 2017; Park et al. 2018; Song et al. 2020)
- 28-day intratracheal instillation studies (Hadrup et al. 2019; Fujita et al. 2023a; Yamashita et al. 2024)
- 90-day and 28-day intratracheal studies in rats (Fujita et al. 2021, 2025a, b)
- 28-day nose-only inhalation exposure in rats (Yamashita et al. 2025)

Table 4.1 Summary of animal studies evaluating the pulmonary effects of nanocellulose materials (NCMs)

ID	Test material	Animal	Administration method	Dose	Post-administration evaluation time	References
1	NFC, Bulk-sized Cellulose fibrils, MWCNTs	Mouse	Oropharyngeal aspiration	10, 40 μg/body	28 days	Ilves et al. (2018)
2	TEMPO-oxidized NFC	Mouse	Oropharyngeal aspiration	10, 40, 80, 200 μg/body	24 h	Catalán et al. (2017)
3	NCF, CNCs, SWCNTs, Crocidolite asbestos	Mouse	Oropharyngeal aspiration	40 μg/body	14 days	Park et al. (2018)
4	NFC, Carboxylated NFCs	Mouse	Intratracheal instillation	6, 18 μg/body	28 days	Hadrup et al. (2019)
5	TEMPO-oxidized CNFs	Mouse	Oropharyngeal aspiration	50 μg/body	3 and 14 days	Song et al. (2020)
6	TEMPO-oxidized CNFs, Mechanically fibrillated CNFs, MWCNTs	Rat	Intratracheal instillation	0.5, 1.0, 2.0 mg/kg	90 days	Fujita et al. (2021)
7	TEMPO-oxidized CNFs, MWCNTs	Mouse	Intratracheal instillation	80 μg/body	28 days	Fujita et al. (2023a)
8	Short mechanically fibrillated CNFs	Mouse	Intratracheal instillation	200 μg/body	28 days	Yamashita et al. (2024)
9	TEMPO-oxidized CNFs, Mechanically fibrillated CNFs, Short mechanically fibrillated CNFs, MWCNTs	Rat	Intratracheal instillation	2.0 mg/kg	28 and 90 days	Fujita et al. (2025a)
10	Mechanically fibrillated CNFs	Rat	Nasal inhalation exposure	1.5, 7, 35 mg/m^3	28 days	Yamashita et al. (2025)
11	TEMPO-oxidized CNFs, Mechanically fibrillated CNFs, CNCs, MWCNTs	Rat	Intratracheal instillation	2.0 mg/kg	28 days	Fujita et al. (2025b)

Abbreviations: NFC (nanofibrillated cellulose) and NCF (nanofibrillar cellulose) are collectively referred to as CNFs (cellulose nanofibrils) throughout this chapter. Doses are reported as described in the original studies and therefore vary according to the exposure method

Key findings from representative studies are summarized below, while detailed descriptions of NEDO project studies are provided in Sect. 4.3.

Ilves et al. (2018) investigated the immunomodulatory effects of four nanofibrillated cellulose (NFC) types using macrophage cell lines and murine respiratory exposure, comparing them with bulk cellulose and rigid MWCNTs. Two NFCs were nonfunctionalized and two were chemically modified. One nonfunctionalized NFC reduced cell viability and induced proinflammatory cytokines in vitro. In vivo, all cellulose materials triggered innate immune responses within 24 h, with nonfunctionalized NFCs additionally inducing Th2-type inflammation. Although immune responses persisted at 28 days, they were markedly attenuated. NFCs were not fully cleared from the lungs within 1 month, indicating biodurability. Compared with MWCNTs, NFCs induced milder effects, but responses were comparable to or exceeded those of bulk cellulose. These findings highlight the influence of surface chemistry and structural properties on NFC bioactivity and support the need for material-specific safety evaluations.

Catalán et al. (2017) assessed the genotoxic and inflammatory effects of TEMPO-oxidized NFCs in mice following single pharyngeal aspiration. DNA damage was detected in lung cells at lower doses (10–80 μg/mouse) after 24 h, whereas no genotoxic effects were observed in BAL cells or bone marrow, suggesting localized pulmonary responses. NFC exposure also induced acute inflammation, evidenced by increased immune cell recruitment and elevated mRNA expression of TNF-α, IL-1β, IL-6, and CXCL5, although corresponding protein levels remained largely unchanged. Histological analyses revealed dose-dependent accumulation of NFCs in the bronchi, alveoli, and macrophages, along with neutrophilic infiltration. These findings indicate that TEMPO-oxidized NFC can induce transient DNA damage and acute inflammatory responses in the lungs, without systemic genotoxicity. However, the study design did not clarify whether these effects persist beyond the acute phase, highlighting the need for further long-term investigations.

Park et al. (2018) investigated pulmonary immune responses in BALB/c mice following oropharyngeal aspiration of CNFs, CNCs, single-walled carbon nanotubes (SWCNTs), and crocidolite asbestos (ASB). By day 14, ASB and SWCNTs induced pronounced inflammation, characterized by elevated immune cell counts and lactate dehydrogenase (LDH) levels. In contrast, CNFs elicited a milder response, with a Th1-type immune polarization distinct from the Th2-like profile associated with ASB. CNCs and SWCNTs produced heterogeneous immune patterns. Cytokine and chemokine expression profiles, as well as antigen presentation markers, varied significantly among materials. These findings highlight the material-specific nature of pulmonary immune modulation and underscore the importance of evaluating immunological outcomes when assessing the safety of fibrous nanomaterials.

Hadrup et al. (2019) examined whether carboxylation could mitigate the pulmonary and systemic toxicity of NFC. Three NFC variants—unmodified FINE NFC, carboxylated NFC [AS(-COOH)], and biocide-containing BIOCID FINE NFC—were administered intratracheally to mice. FINE NFC induced neutrophil influx in bronchoalveolar lavage fluid and elevated serum SAA3 levels, indicating acute inflammation. In contrast, AS(-COOH) elicited significantly weaker responses, suggesting that carboxylation reduces toxicity, potentially by modifying the surface hydroxyl (-OH) groups involved in inflammatory signaling. DNA damage was observed across all materials, doses, and time points. The presence of biocide BIM

MC4901 did not account for the reduced toxicity, as BIOCID FINE NFC showed similar effects to FINE NFC. These findings highlight surface chemistry as a key determinant of NFC bioactivity and support carboxylation as a strategy for safer material design.

Song et al. (2020) investigated pulmonary inflammation and transcriptomic changes induced by CNFs in female C57BL/6 mice following oropharyngeal aspiration. Marked inflammatory gene expression was observed at 3 days postexposure, accompanied by differential expression of 201 genes—primarily related to immune and inflammatory pathways, including chemokines, NK cell receptors, CD antigens, and interferon-induced proteins. By day 14, gene expression changes were substantially reduced (35 genes affected), suggesting recovery of pulmonary homeostasis. These findings demonstrate that CNFs can elicit acute but potentially reversible inflammatory and immunogenomic responses in the lungs. Overall, the study provides mechanistic insights into CNF-induced pulmonary effects and supports the need for transcriptomic profiling in nanotoxicology risk assessment.

Stoudmann et al. (2020) emphasized that scientific understanding of CNF inhalation effects remains incomplete, particularly with respect to biopersistence following internalization. They highlighted the need for chronic low-dose exposure studies and reinforced the importance of workplace exposure controls and protective measures during NCMNanocellulose material (NCM) processing.

Similarly, Shatkin et al. (2016) identified inhalation exposure as the primary occupational concern for NCMsNanocellulose materials (NCMs) and highlighted gaps in chronic toxicity data, clearance kinetics, and standardized testing protocols. Addressing these gaps is essential for developing safety data sheets (SDS) compliant with globally harmonized system (GHS) and ensuring safe commercialization. In Japan, the NEDO projects (FY2017–2019 and FY2020–2024) have generated additional data on pulmonary inflammation, pulmonary distribution and retention, macrophage phagocytosis, and in vitro cytotoxicity (Sai and Fujita 2020; Fujita and Moriyama 2025). These studies are discussed in detail in Sect. 4.3.

Multiple animal studies investigating the inhalation toxicity of CNCs have been reported. An overview of representative studies is provided below and summarized in Table 4.2.

Joseph et al. (2021) investigated pulmonary toxicity and transcriptomic alterations following whole-body inhalation exposure to CNCs in rats (20 mg/m^3, 6 h/day for 14 days). CNC exposure significantly increased LDH activity, proinflammatory cytokine levels, oxidant production, and macrophage and neutrophil counts in bronchoalveolar lavage fluid, accompanied by mild histopathological changes. RNA sequencing identified 531 differentially expressed genes, with enrichment in inflammation- and oxidative stress-related pathways, including leukocyte trafficking, complement activation, interleukin-10 (IL-10) signaling, and nuclear factor erythroid 2–related factor 2 (NRF2)-mediated responses. These findings indicate that CNCs induce lung toxicity primarily through inflammatory and oxidative mechanisms, providing molecular insight into potential health risks and underscoring the importance of mechanistic evaluation in nanomaterial safety assessment.

Table 4.2 Summary of animal studies evaluating the pulmonary effects of cellulose nanocrystals (CNCs)

ID	Test material	Animal	Administration method	Dose	Observation period	References
1	CNCs	Rat	Whole-body inhalation exposure	20 mg/m^3, 6 h/day	14 days	Joseph et al. (2021)
2	CNCS (gel/suspension), CNCP (powder)	Mouse	Oropharyngeal aspiration	50, 100, 200 μg/body	24 h	Yanamala et al. (2014)
3	CNCs	Mouse	Oropharyngeal aspiration	40 μg/body, twice/week for 3 weeks	90 days	Farcas et al. (2016)
4	CNCs	Mouse	Oropharyngeal aspiration	40 μg/body, twice/week for 3 weeks	90 days	Shvedova et al. (2016)
5	CNCs, TEMPO-oxidized CNFs, Mechanically fibrillated CNFs, MWCNTs	Rat	Intratracheal instillation	2.0 mg/kg	28 days	Fujita et al. (2025b)

Yanamala et al. (2014) evaluated the pulmonary immunotoxicity of two CNC forms—gel/suspension (CNCS) and powder (CNCP)—in C57BL/6 mice following pharyngeal aspiration. Both forms induced innate inflammatory responses, as evidenced by increased leukocyte and eosinophil counts in bronchoalveolar lavage fluid. CNCP exposure resulted in greater tissue damage, whereas CNCS exposure led to significant accumulation of oxidatively modified proteins and elevated inflammatory cytokine expression. Notably, CNCP particles were morphologically longer than CNCS, suggesting that particle size and shape critically influence biological responses. These findings underscore the importance of evaluating CNC toxicity in relation to physicochemical properties, particularly given that different processing methods yield structurally distinct NCMs.

Farcas et al. (2016) investigated the long-term reproductive toxicity of CNCs in male mice following repeated pharyngeal aspiration. Three months after exposure, CNCs significantly impaired sperm concentration, motility, morphology, and DNA integrity. These effects were associated with elevated testicular proinflammatory cytokines, increased myeloperoxidase activity, and oxidative stress in the testes and epididymis. Histopathological analysis revealed interstitial edema, degeneration of seminiferous tubules, and arrested spermatogenesis. Hormonal imbalances were also observed, including disrupted levels of testosterone and luteinizing hormone. These findings suggest that pulmonary exposure to CNCs can induce sustained adverse effects on male reproductive function, highlighting the importance of evaluating systemic outcomes in nanocellulose safety assessments.

Shvedova et al. (2016) examined sex-specific pulmonary responses to repeated exposure to respirable CNCs in C57BL/6 mice. Following pharyngeal aspiration (40 μg/mouse, twice weekly for 3 weeks), both male and female mice exhibited lung inflammation, oxidative stress, elevated transforming growth factor beta (TGF-β) and collagen levels, and impaired pulmonary function. Notably, female mice displayed significantly more pronounced pathological and transcriptomic changes, including enhanced cytokine and chemokine expression and distinct mRNA expression profiles. These findings highlight potential sex-based differences in susceptibility to CNC-induced pulmonary toxicity and underscore the importance of incorporating sex as a biological variable in nanotoxicological risk assessment.

Collectively, the available animal studies indicate that CNCs can induce pulmonary inflammation, oxidative stress, and alterations in immune responses, with some studies also reporting systemic effects, including reproductive toxicity and sex-dependent differences in susceptibility. The magnitude and nature of these responses appear to depend on physicochemical characteristics, exposure conditions, and biological factors. However, important uncertainties remain regarding long-term retention, chronic toxicity, and potential systemic translocation following inhalation exposure. Further low-dose, long-term inhalation studies are needed to clarify the biodurability and long-term health implications of CNC exposure.

Beyond inflammatory and toxicological outcomes, emerging evidence suggests that some NCMs may also modulate immune function. Čolić et al. (2020) evaluated the immunological effects of nanocellulose—particularly CNFs and CNCs—and demonstrated their potential to induce immune tolerance. This phenomenon, characterized by suppression of excessive immune activation and inflammation, suggests possible applications in wound healing and tissue regeneration. However, it remains unclear whether such immunomodulatory effects are sustained under long-term exposure conditions.

Finally, systematic validation of correlations between in vitro and in vivo responses is required to improve the predictive value of toxicological models. Such efforts are essential for establishing comprehensive safety profiles for NCMs and for guiding the responsible development and commercialization of NCM-based products.

4.2.3 In Vitro Studies of NCMs

Several in vitro studies have evaluated the pulmonary toxicity of NCMs, including CNFs and CNCs, using alveolar epithelial cells, macrophages, and other relevant cell models. A549 alveolar epithelial cells and THP-1-derived macrophages have been among the most commonly used systems for assessing cytotoxic, inflammatory, oxidative stress–related, and genotoxic responses (Menas et al. 2017; Pinto et al. 2022; Yanamala et al. 2016; Bhattacharya et al. 2017). Key findings from representative studies are summarized in Table 4.3, while detailed descriptions of NEDO project studies are provided in Sect. 4.3.

Table 4.3 Summary of representative in vitro studies evaluating the biological effects of CNFs and CNCs

ID	Test material	Cell type	Exposure duration	Exposure concentration	Endpoints	References
1	CNCs, NCF	A549	24, 72 h	1.5, 15, 45 μg/cm^2	Cytotoxicity, Oxidative Stress, Cytokines	Menas et al. (2017)
2	CMFS, CNFS, CNCs	A549	24 h	1.5, 3, 6, 12.5, 25, 50 μg/cm^2	Cellular Uptake, Cytotoxicity, Genotoxicity	Pinto et al. (2022)
3	Various CNF-containing Cellulose Nanomaterials	A549, THP-1	24, 72 h	<300 μg/mL	Cytotoxicity, Membrane damage, Cytokines	Yanamala et al. (2016)
4	CNFs	THP-1	24, 48 h	<100 μg/mL	Cytotoxicity, Cytokines	Bhattacharya et al. (2017)
5	Unmodified and Modified NFCs	HDF, MRC-5, THP-1	24 h	50–500 μg/mL	Cytotoxicity, ROS, Cytokines, Intracellular observation	Lopes et al. (2017)
6	Unmodified and Modified CNFs	BEAS-2B	24 h	4–1000 μg/mL	Cytotoxicity, ROS, Intracellular observation	Aimonen et al. (2022)
7	TEMPO-oxidized CNFs, Mechanically fibrillated CNFs	MeT-5A, A549, HaCaT, Caco-2, THP-1, NR8383	24 h	2.6, 26 μg/mL	Cytotoxicity, Cytokines	Horie et al. (2023)
8	TEMPO-oxidized CNFs, Phosphorylated CNFs, Mechanically fibrillated CNFs, Citrus CNFs, ACC-method CNFs, Standard CNCs, sulfuric acid-hydrolyzed CNCs, desulfurized CNCs	NR8383	24, 48 h	100 μg/mL	Cytotoxicity, ROS, Cytokines, Intracellular observation, Comprehensive gene expression analysis	Fujita et al. (2025b, c)

Abbreviations: NFC (nanofibrillated cellulose) and NCF (nanofibrillar cellulose) are collectively referred to as CNFs (cellulose nanofibrils) throughout this chapter. Exposure concentrations are reported as described in the original studies and therefore vary according to the test system and exposure metric

Menas et al. (2017) compared the cytotoxic and immunological effects of CNCs and nanofibrillated cellulose (NCF) using human lung epithelial A549 cells exposed to five nanocellulose types for 24 and 72 h. NCF induced stronger cytotoxicity and oxidative stress, whereas CNCs elicited a more pronounced inflammatory response, characterized by elevated cytokine and chemokine secretion. Notably, CNC particles were internalized by cells, whereas NCF was not. Cytokine clustering analysis revealed that NCF elicited response profiles similar to carbon nanofibers, while CNCs showed patterns resembling those induced by chitin, a known immunomodulator. These findings highlight the importance of morphology and surface chemistry in determining cellular uptake and biological responses and emphasize the need for material-specific safety evaluation.

Pinto et al. (2022) evaluated the cytotoxicity and genotoxicity of cellulose micro/nanomaterials (CMNMs)—including cellulose microfibrils (CMFs), CNFs, and CNCs—in A549 cells, using MWCNTs as reference materials. Transmission electron microscopy (TEM) revealed cellular uptake of all CMNMs except CNCs. While CMNMs did not induce cytotoxicity, CMFs significantly increased micronucleus frequency, indicating genotoxic potential independent of oxidative DNA damage. In contrast, CNFs and CNCs showed no genotoxic effects. These results demonstrate that biological responses vary by particle type and structure, emphasizing the need for alternative genotoxicity endpoints and mechanistic studies.

Yanamala et al. (2016) examined biological responses to various NCMs in A549 cells and THP-1 macrophage-like cells. A549 cells exhibited minimal cytotoxicity, whereas THP-1 cells showed pronounced cytotoxic and inflammatory responses, particularly following exposure to CNCs and lignin-coated CNFs. Hierarchical clustering analysis identified NCM-specific response profiles and key inflammatory mediators, although no clear correlation between surface properties and cytotoxic outcomes was observed. These findings emphasize cell type-specific sensitivity and support the use of multicellular models in NCM safety evaluation.

Bhattacharya et al. (2017) conducted cytokine profiling using THP-1 macrophages to assess the immunotoxic potential of 19 engineered nanomaterials (ENMs), including NCMs. CNFs were noncytotoxic at concentrations up to 100 μg/mL but induced potent inflammatory responses at subcytotoxic concentrations, comparable to those observed for TiO_2 and CeO_2 nanoparticles. Pathway analysis revealed distinct ENM groupings based on activation or suppression of peroxisome proliferator-activated receptor (PPAR) and liver X receptor/retinoid X receptor (LXR/RXR) nuclear receptor pathways. These results suggest that NCMs may exert immunomodulatory effects in the absence of overt cytotoxicity, underscoring the importance of mechanistic profiling.

Lopes et al. (2017) examined human dermal fibroblasts, lung epithelial cells (MRC-5), and THP-1 macrophages exposed to wood-derived NFC gels, either unmodified or surface-modified (carboxymethylated or hydroxypropyltrimethylammonium-modified). None of the NFC variants induced cytotoxicity or reactive oxygen species (ROS) production. However, unmodified NFCs triggered proinflammatory responses in THP-1 cells, as evidenced by the elevated TNF-α and IL-1β expression, whereas surface-modified NFCs did not.

TEM analyses revealed differences in fibril dispersion and agglomeration depending on surface chemistry. These findings indicate that surface functionalization can modulate immune responses and support design strategies aimed at improving biocompatibility.

Aimonen et al. (2022) investigated the genotoxic potential of CNFs in human bronchial epithelial BEAS-2B cells, focusing on surface chemistry and fibril size. Three size fractions (fine, medium, and coarse) of four CNF types—unmodified, TEMPO-oxidized, carboxymethylated, and cationically modified—were evaluated. No significant cytotoxicity was observed; however, several CNFs induced ROS production, and two formulations (fine E-CNF and coarse C-CNF) caused DNA strand breaks and chromosomal damage, likely mediated by ROS. These results demonstrate that both surface functionalization and fibril size influence genotoxic outcomes and reinforce the need for case-by-case evaluation.

Key Takeaways Collectively, the available in vitro studies indicate that NCMs generally exhibit low cytotoxicity across a range of cell models. However, inflammatory responses, immunomodulatory effects, oxidative stress, and occasional genotoxic signals have been reported depending on material characteristics and experimental conditions. Surface chemistry, particle size, morphology, and cell type are important determinants of biological responses. These findings support the use of integrated testing strategies that combine mechanistic approaches with OECD-compliant in vivo studies to improve hazard identification and risk assessment of NCMs.

4.3 Key Findings from the NEDO Project

4.3.1 Evaluation of Inhalation Effects of NCMs via Intratracheal Instillation Studies

Under the NEDO projects (FY2017–2019 and FY2020–2024), the National Institute of Advanced Industrial Science and Technology (AIST), in collaboration with industry partners, developed standardized preparation methods for NCMs and conducted comprehensive characterization studies to evaluate inhalation-related effects. Toxicity assessments were primarily performed using intratracheal instillation tests in rats, and the outcomes were compiled in a Japanese-language manual published in 2020, as well as in the English publication *A Manual for Toxicity Testing of Cellulose Nanofibers* (Fujita et al. 2023a). In the subsequent project phase, efforts shifted toward the development and validation of simple and rapid evaluation methods for inhalation effects that minimize or replace animal testing, aiming to enable assessment across a broader range of NCM types, including both CNFs and CNCs.

Inhalation toxicity is conventionally evaluated using whole-body or nose-only inhalation exposure studies in rodents, as specified in OECD TGs (Kasai et al.

2016). However, these studies require large-scale facilities, advanced aerosol generation systems, and continuous real-time control of exposure concentrations, rendering them costly and technically demanding. As a result, this approach is often impractical for routine evaluation of multiple NCM types. Conversely, intratracheal instillation—wherein a liquid dispersion of the test material is directly administered into the trachea—offers several practical advantages. These include simpler equipment requirements, reduced test material consumption, and, most importantly, precise control of the lung-deposited dose. This accurate dosing capability enables reproducible and comparative evaluations under identical conditions, which is particularly valuable for elucidating the relationship between material properties and biological responses and for generating scientific evidence relevant to product development and risk assessment.

Consequently, intratracheal instillation has been widely used as a practical alternative approach for hazard screening and comparative assessment of engineered nanomaterials. Previous studies from our group and others have demonstrated the utility of this method for evaluating pulmonary responses to fibrous and particulate nanomaterials (Honda et al. 2017; Fujita et al. 2009a, b, 2010, 2015a, b, 2016). Nevertheless, during the initial NEDO project (FY2017–2019), reports on NCM instillation studies were limited to a single 28-day study in mice (Hadrup et al. 2019).

Intratracheal instillation involves administration of a bolus dose of liquid-dispersed material directly into the trachea, and toxicity is evaluated based on subsequent biological responses, such as pulmonary inflammation. This approach differs fundamentally from inhalation exposure studies, in which animals inhale airborne materials over time, and therefore requires careful experimental design and interpretation. Because instillation delivers a concentrated dose at a single time point, it may elicit biological responses that differ from those caused by realistic inhalation exposure due to localized overexposure, commonly referred to as the "bolus effect." Accordingly, careful attention must be paid to test material preparation and dose selection. When administering NCMs via intratracheal instillation, it is essential to prepare stable dispersions—whether as slurries or powders—that preserve the intrinsic physicochemical properties of the materials. In addition, thorough characterization of dispersion behavior and biological activity of NCMs is critical for accurate interpretation of inhalation toxicity potential. To evaluate the distribution and retention of NCMs in the lungs following instillation, reliable methods for extracting and analyzing NCMs from lung tissue must be established.

To address these challenges, the NEDO projects focused on the development of standardized intratracheal instillation protocols for NCMs, thereby contributing to the international harmonization of nanomaterial safety testing. The overall workflow developed through the NEDO projects is summarized in Fig. 4.1. These efforts represent an important step toward integrating physicochemical characterization with biological endpoints and advancing alternative assessment approaches that reduce reliance on animal testing, in alignment with OECD and ISO frameworks.

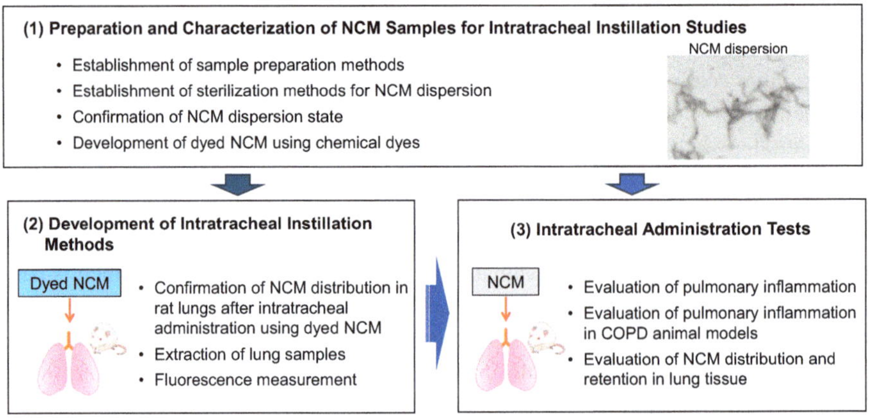

Fig. 4.1 A flowchart depicting the development of standardized intratracheal instillation testing methods for nanocellulose materials (NCMs)

4.3.1.1 Preparation and Characterization of NCM Samples for Intratracheal Instillation Studies

To ensure reliable intratracheal instillation studies, standardized procedures for the preparation of NCM dispersions were established within the NEDO projects. Because NCMs can exhibit agglomeration, sedimentation, and viscosity-dependent dispersion behavior, stable and reproducible dispersions are essential for meaningful toxicity evaluation. Accordingly, preparation conditions were optimized according to material characteristics and study objectives to minimize variability and ensure consistent dosing.

Comprehensive physicochemical characterization was conducted in parallel with sample preparation to support dose selection and interpretation of biological responses. The absolute dry concentration of NCMs was determined in accordance with the Japanese Industrial Standards (JIS) P 8203:2010. In addition, parameters potentially relevant to inhalation toxicity—including viscosity, pH, zeta potential, fiber diameter, and fiber length—were systematically evaluated.

Because NCMs are derived from natural wood pulp, there is a potential risk of microbial contamination in aqueous dispersions prepared for biological testing. Accordingly, biological characterization was also performed, including quantitative analyses of total bacteria, fungi, endotoxins, and β-glucans. Although microbial control is essential in animal studies, the use of chemical sterilization methods is limited due to their potential interference with material properties. To address this issue, gamma irradiation was employed as a nonthermal, nonchemical approach for microbial inactivation. Irradiation doses of 0.5, 1, 5, and 10 kGy were evaluated. At 10 kGy, a significant reduction in fiber length was observed, whereas doses of 0.5–1 kGy had minimal effects on physicochemical properties while providing sufficient inactivation of bacteria and fungi (Ogura et al. 2025; Horie et al. 2023). These findings support the use of low-dose gamma irradiation as a practical sterilization method for NCM toxicity studies while preserving key physicochemical characteristics.

In intratracheal instillation studies, it is also important to confirm whether the administered material is evenly distributed within the lungs. However, NCMs are optically transparent, making direct visualization in tissue sections difficult. To overcome this limitation, the NEDO project (FY2017–2019) developed a novel approach using chemically dyed NCMs to enable quantitative evaluation of in vivo retention and pulmonary distribution. Dyes were selected to minimize interference with tissue background and to ensure strong binding to NCMs. Using this method, the distribution and residual amounts of NCMs in individual lung lobes could be quantitatively evaluated, providing important information on pulmonary deposition and retention following administration (Fujita et al. 2020, 2023b, 2025a). Details of this methodology are provided in Sect. 4.3.1.3.4.

Collectively, these efforts established a standardized framework for NCM preparation, characterization, sterilization, and pulmonary tracking, providing a robust foundation for the intratracheal instillation studies described in the following sections.

4.3.1.2 Development of an Intratracheal Instillation Method for NCMs

In intratracheal instillation studies, test materials are administered directly into the trachea of animals using dedicated delivery devices. Depending on the viscosity or irritant properties of the test material, animals may experience transient respiratory distress or abnormal behavior immediately after administration, potentially confounding the interpretation of toxicological outcomes. Because NCM dispersions often exhibit relatively high viscosity, they may also be difficult to expel from the instillation device and may not distribute uniformly within lung tissue.

To address these challenges, a method was developed to preassess the concentration of NCM dispersions and their injectability through the delivery device (Fujita et al. 2020, 2023b). As part of this refinement, injectability of phosphorylated NCM dispersions was evaluated using a metallic oral probe, which is commonly employed in toxicity studies. Dispersions at concentrations of 4, 5, and 6 mg/mL were prepared by diluting a 20 mg/mL stock solution with distilled water. Each dispersion was loaded into a syringe fitted with an oral probe, and the ejection behavior was examined by measuring the distance traveled by the expelled material from the probe tip, using distilled water as a reference.

As shown in Fig. 4.2, dispersions with concentrations exceeding 4 mg/mL exhibited reduced ejection performance due to increased viscosity and thixotropic behavior, which may impair uniform pulmonary distribution. Based on these findings, 4.0 mg/mL was identified as the optimal upper concentration for phosphorylated NCMs in intratracheal instillation studies. Importantly, preliminary administration tests in experimental animals are also required to observe potential adverse effects, such as suffocation or abnormal behavior. Such observations are critical for determining safe and appropriate dose ranges for NCM dispersions. Overall, the described

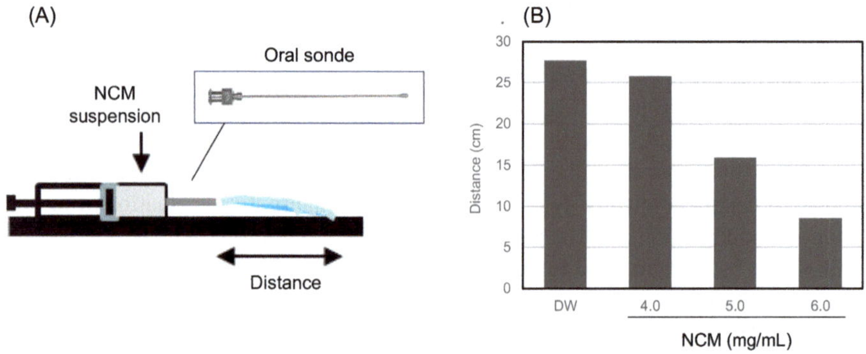

Fig. 4.2 Evaluation of the injectability of NCMs using a metallic oral probe. (**A**) Schematic illustration of the experimental setup used to assess the ejection performance of NCM dispersions. Test dispersions were loaded into a syringe fitted with a metallic oral probe, and the distance traveled by the expelled liquid from the probe tip was measured as an indicator of injectability. (**B**) Ejection distances of phosphorylated NCM dispersions at concentrations of 4.0, 5.0, and 6.0 mg/mL, compared with distilled water. Ejection distance decreased with increasing NCM concentration, indicating reduced injectability due to increased viscosity and thixotropic behavior. Ejection distance decreased markedly at concentrations above 4.0 mg/mL

method provides a practical approach for preassessing both the physical injectability and biological tolerability of NCM dispersions, thereby contributing to the refinement and reliability of inhalation toxicity studies.

4.3.1.3 Intratracheal Instillation Study

4.3.1.3.1 Pulmonary Inflammation Assessment Over 90 Days Following Intratracheal Instillation

As a preliminary step, NCM dispersions were intratracheally instilled into rats to evaluate formulation tolerability and to confirm the absence of acute adverse effects associated with the instillation procedure itself. Animals were monitored for several days after administration to assess general health status. In parallel, key formulation parameters, including dispersion viscosity and particle concentration, were examined to establish preparation conditions suitable for intratracheal instillation and to define acceptable dose ranges.

Based on these preliminary evaluations, a main study was conducted in which three types of NCMs, together with multi-walled carbon nanotubes (MWCNTs) as a comparative reference material, were intratracheally administered at doses of 0.5, 1.0, and 2.0 mg/kg. Pulmonary inflammation and related biological responses were then systematically evaluated over a 90-day observation period.

MWCNTs were selected as a reference material due to their well-documented biopersistence and strong inflammation-inducing potential, as demonstrated in previous toxicological studies (Murphy et al. 2011). This comparison enabled evaluation of NCM-induced inflammatory responses relative to a fibrous nanomaterial with established pulmonary toxicity. In addition, our research group has accumulated extensive experience with MWCNTs through prior intratracheal instillation and in vitro studies, ensuring consistency and reliability in comparative assessments (Fujita et al. 2016, 2020).

Among the NCMs tested, TEMPO-oxidized and phosphorylated CNFs—characterized by similar fiber diameter and length distributions—induced inflammatory responses in the alveolar region shortly after instillation; however, these responses subsided by day 90. In contrast, mechanically fibrillated CNFs derived from softwood bleached kraft pulp were predominantly deposited around the terminal bronchioles, where relatively thick and long fibers were observed (Fig. 4.3). Although this CNF type also elicited acute inflammatory responses in the alveoli, the severity was lower than that observed with phosphorylated and TEMPO-oxidized CNFs, and inflammation had resolved by the end of the observation period. In comparison, MWCNTs induced persistent and severe pulmonary inflammation throughout the 90-day period, with no evidence of resolution. Hierarchical cluster analysis of gene expression profiles revealed that the three NCMs exhibited broadly similar expression patterns, whereas the profile of MWCNTs was markedly distinct.

These findings suggest that pulmonary inflammation induced by NCMs is influenced by fiber diameter and length distribution, and that their inflammatory potential is substantially lower than that of MWCNTs (Fujita et al. 2021). One factor contributing to NCM deposition in the alveoli and terminal bronchioles is their nano- to submicron-scale dimensions, which approximates the aerodynamic characteristics of respirable dust as defined by ISO 7708 (ISO 1995), with a 50% cut-off at 4 μm. In rodent studies, particles with a mass median aerodynamic diameter (MMAD) greater than 5–10 μm have been reported to exhibit limited deposition in the alveolar region (Yamato 1994). In contrast, due to their small dimensions, NCMs are more likely to reach the deep lung, unlike conventional cellulose particles that are more efficiently cleared by mucociliary transport.

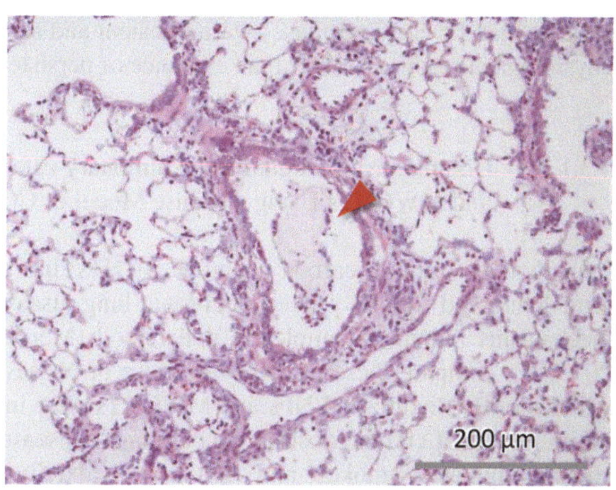

Fig. 4.3 Histological section of rat lung showing deposition of mechanically fibrillated CNFs around a terminal bronchiole at Day 1 after intratracheal instillation. The red arrow indicates CNF deposits localized within the bronchiolar lumen. Hematoxylin and eosin staining. Scale bar = 200 μm

It should be noted that these observations are based on intratracheal instillation studies, in which NCMs were dispersed in liquid and directly administered to animals. Under actual exposure conditions, NCM morphology may vary substantially depending on droplet size and drying behavior in the air. In general, droplets larger than several tens of micrometers settle rapidly due to gravity, whereas smaller droplets evaporate quickly. Consequently, when aqueous NCM dispersions are sprayed, dried agglomerates may become airborne and potentially inhalable (Chap. 7). Studies examining droplets generated from NCM dispersions have shown that dried particles appear as solid agglomerates, whereas network-like NCM structures are observed in droplets captured without drying (Ogura et al. 2020). Furthermore, under conditions of very high humidity that inhibit evaporation, or when droplets are generated from slowly evaporating media such as oils, exposure to fibrous NCMs in their dispersed state may occur. These findings underscore the need for further investigations to clarify NCM morphology and behavior during inhalation of sprayed dispersions under realistic exposure scenarios.

4.3.1.3.2 Evaluation of Inhalation Effects of Mechanically Fibrillated CNFs: 28-day Intratracheal Instillation Study in Mice

Under the NEDO project (FY2020–2024), the University of Fukui conducted a single-dose, 28-day intratracheal instillation study in male C57BL/6JJmsSlc mice to evaluate the inhalation effects of short-fiber mechanically fibrillated CNFs (average fiber length: ~500 nm; average fiber diameter: ~45 nm), using a dose of 0.2 mg/body (Yamashita et al. 2024).

No mortality occurred in either the control or CNF-treated groups during the observation period. On Day 3 postinstillation, transient changes were observed, including body weight loss, a significant increase in eosinophil counts, a significant decrease in reticulocyte counts, and increased lung weight. However, all observed changes resolved over time, and no significant abnormalities in hematological parameters or histopathological findings were observed on Day 28. These findings indicate that the early responses were transient and are best interpreted as adaptive physiological reactions rather than evidence of persistent adverse effects.

4.3.1.3.3 Comparative Evaluation of Pulmonary Effects of CNFs and MWCNTs Using a Mouse Model of COPD

Inhalation exposure to carbon nanotubes (CNTs) has been associated with airway remodeling and fibrosis related to chronic lung diseases, although the underlying mechanisms remain incompletely understood (Mercer et al. 2011; Porter et al. 2010). To compare these effects with those of NCMs, a study was conducted in which TEMPO-oxidized CNFs and MWCNTs were intratracheally instilled into a mouse model of chronic obstructive pulmonary disease (COPD) induced by mainstream cigarette smoke, and inhalation toxicity was evaluated 28 days

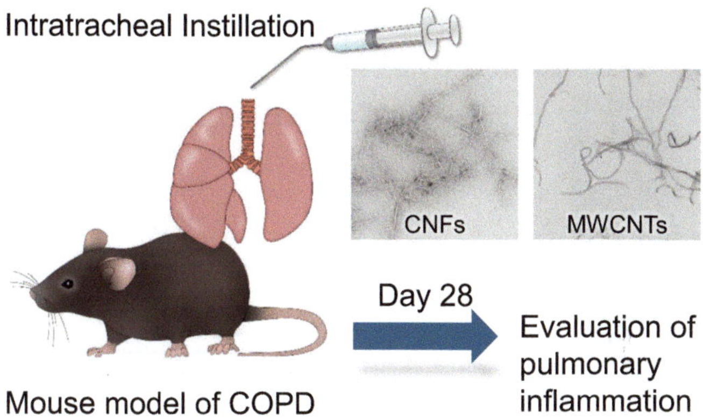

Fig. 4.4 Comparative evaluation of the pulmonary effects of CNFs and MWCNTs in a mouse model of COPD. TEMPO-oxidized CNFs or MWCNTs were administered by intratracheal instillation to mice with cigarette smoke–induced COPD. Pulmonary inflammation and related biological responses were evaluated at Day 28 after administration

postinstillation (Fig. 4.4) (Fujita et al. 2023b). In the group administered 80 μg of TEMPO-oxidized CNFs per animal, no significant changes were observed on Day 28 in lung histopathology, BALF cellularity, or inflammatory cytokine levels. These findings suggest that CNFs do not strongly exacerbate pulmonary inflammation and may not interfere with recovery from cigarette smoke-induced inflammatory responses. In contrast, mice treated with MWCNTs at the same dose exhibited pronounced histopathological alterations, increased BALF cellularity, and elevated inflammatory cytokine levels on Day 28. Collectively, these results indicate that CNFs induce substantially milder pulmonary effects than MWCNTs in a mouse model of COPD and do not hinder recovery from cigarette smoke-induced lung inflammation.

4.3.1.3.4 Evaluation of Pulmonary Inflammation and Persistence of CNFs

Pulmonary inflammation at 28 days following intratracheal instillation was evaluated using three types of CNFs: TEMPO-oxidized CNFs, mechanically fibrillated CNFs derived from bleached softwood kraft pulp, and short-length mechanically fibrillated CNFs (Fujita et al. 2025a). To assess the potential contribution of endotoxin contamination in CNF suspensions, a comparative study was conducted using lipopolysaccharide (LPS) administration. The results indicated that TEMPO-oxidized CNFs induced mild alveolar inflammation, mechanically fibrillated CNFs from bleached softwood kraft pulp induced granuloma formation, and short-length mechanically fibrillated CNFs elicited both inflammatory responses and granuloma formation.

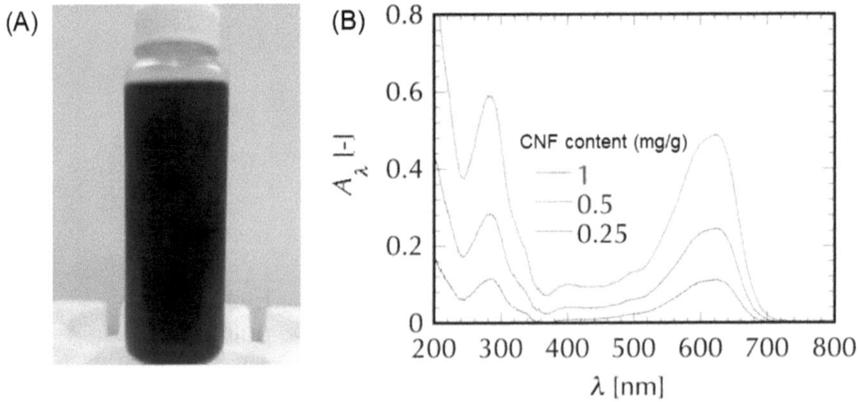

Fig. 4.5 Spectrophotometric characterization of dyed CNF dispersions. (**A**) Dyed CNF dispersion prepared using a dark blue reactive dye. (**B**) Absorption spectra of dyed CNF dispersions at concentrations of 0.25, 0.5, and 1.0 mg/g. Characteristic absorption peaks were observed in the visible range, particularly around 610–630 nm. Absorbance increased with increasing CNF concentration, enabling spectrophotometric quantification

Analysis of BALF revealed distinct response profiles. TEMPO-oxidized CNFs increased leukocyte and macrophage counts, mechanically fibrillated CNFs from bleached softwood kraft pulp increased total protein levels, and short-length CNFs markedly increased neutrophil counts and proinflammatory cytokines, including MIP-1α, IL-1β, and IL-18. In contrast, LPS administration induced only minimal responses, indicating that endotoxin contamination in CNF suspensions had a limited contribution to the observed pulmonary responses.

To enable accurate tracking and quantification of CNFs within lung tissue, a dyed CNF dispersion was developed using a dark blue reactive dye. The dyed CNFs exhibited characteristic absorption in the visible range (610–630 nm), enabling spectrophotometric quantification (Fig. 4.5). A linear relationship between absorbance at 616 nm and CNF concentration was confirmed, ensuring reliable quantitative analysis. The dyed CNFs were further characterized in terms of rheological and morphological properties, including TEM-based fiber length distribution analysis. This labeling approach significantly improved detection sensitivity and enabled robust assessment of CNF persistence and distribution in biological tissues, providing a valuable tool for inhalation toxicity studies.

Information regarding the degradation and persistence of CNFs in the lungs remains limited. Because CNFs are optically transparent, they are difficult to identify in tissue sections using conventional histological methods. To overcome this limitation, a novel method combining chemically prestained CNFs with an extraction protocol incorporating ultrasonication and enzymatic digestion was developed. Spectrophotometric analysis of the extracted stained CNFs enabled accurate tracking and quantification within lung tissue, yielding highly reliable data on material retention (Fujita et al. 2025a).

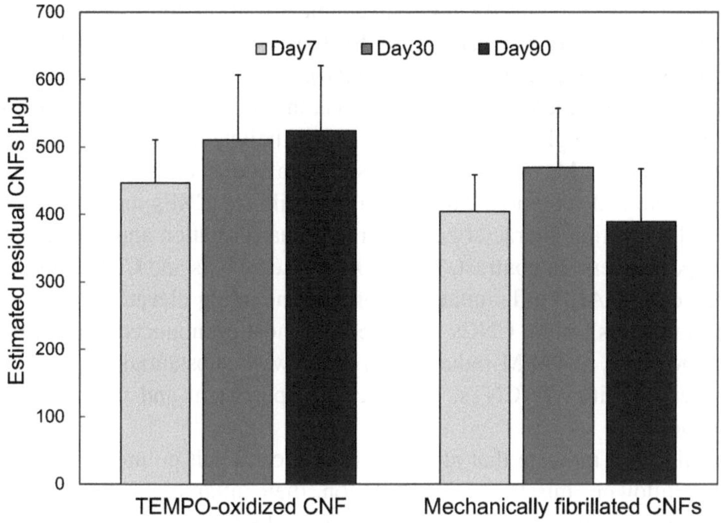

Fig. 4.6 Time-course changes in estimated residual levels of CNFs in rat lung tissue following intratracheal instillation. Estimated residual amounts of TEMPO-oxidized CNFs and mechanically fibrillated CNFs were quantified in lung tissue at Days 7, 30, and 90 after administration using a dye-based extraction and spectrophotometric analysis method. Both CNF types remained detectable in the lung throughout the 90-day observation period

In a 90-day follow-up study, both TEMPO-oxidized CNFs and mechanically fibrillated CNFs evaluated in this study were shown to persist in the lungs over the long term (Fig. 4.6). TEM analysis further confirmed the presence of CNFs within alveolar macrophages, indicating cellular uptake and retention. These findings suggest that CNF degradation in the lungs is extremely slow and that CNFs may accumulate following prolonged or repeated exposure (Fujita et al. 2025a).

Differences in CNF fiber diameter and length were also found to influence pulmonary deposition patterns and inflammatory responses, highlighting the importance of these physicochemical characteristics as key determinants of long-term biological effects. Based on these observations, further long-term studies—particularly under conditions of chronic low-dose exposure are needed to better characterize CNF persistence and its relationship to pulmonary inflammation and other potential adverse outcomes.

4.3.1.3.5 Evaluation of Pulmonary Inflammation and Immune Responses of NCMs

With the increasing industrial and biomedical applications of NCMs, including CNFs and CNCs, concerns have arisen regarding potential inhalation exposure due to their respirable particle size (<10 μm). To investigate pulmonary and immunotoxic effects, a comparative study was conducted using three representative materials—TEMPO-oxidized CNFs, mechanically fibrillated CNFs, and CNCs—with MWCNTs serving as a benchmark for fibrous nanomaterials with well-established pulmonary toxicity (Fujita et al. 2025b).

All materials were administered to rats via intratracheal instillation at a dose of 2.0 mg/kg body weight. At 28 days postinstillation, histopathological analysis revealed that all NCMs were phagocytosed by alveolar macrophages, confirming cellular uptake and retention. Mechanically fibrillated CNFs induced limited pulmonary inflammation characterized by granuloma formation and minimal changes in BALF parameters. In contrast, TEMPO-oxidized CNFs and CNCs induced similar increases in BALF inflammatory markers, including elevated cytokine levels. Among the NCMs tested, CNCs produced the most pronounced histopathological changes; however, all NCM-induced responses were substantially less severe than those observed with MWCNTs, which caused persistent and marked pulmonary inflammation.

These findings indicate that although NCMs can elicit pulmonary and immune responses following intratracheal instillation, their inflammatory potential is considerably lower than that of MWCNTs. The results further underscore the importance of physicochemical properties—such as fiber morphology and surface chemistry—in determining the magnitude and nature of pulmonary responses. Additional studies addressing chronic low-dose exposure and long-term immunological outcomes are needed to support comprehensive risk assessment and regulatory decision-making.

4.3.2 Inhalation Exposure Studies for Evaluating the Inhalation Effects of NCMs

Under the NEDO project (FY2020–2024), the University of Fukui developed and characterized sample preparation methods for inhalation toxicity assessment of NCMs and conducted a rat inhalation exposure study in accordance with OECD TG 412 (OECD 2018a). In this study, mechanically fibrillated CNFs (fib-CNFs) were selected as a representative material, and rats were exposed via nose-only inhalation for 6 h per day over a 28-day period (Yamashita et al. 2025). Exposure concentrations were set at three levels: high (35 mg/m^3), medium (7 mg/m^3), and low (1.5 mg/m^3).

No significant differences were observed between fib-CNF-exposed and control groups in terms of body weight, hematological parameters, or biochemical indices. Histopathological examination of lung tissue revealed increased numbers of macrophages in the alveoli and lung-associated lymph nodes in the fib-CNF exposure groups, accompanied by a significant increase in lung weight. These effects were most pronounced in the high-concentration group, whereas the low-concentration group exhibited only mild inflammatory responses. Based on these findings, the NOAEL for fib-CNFs under the conditions of this 28-day inhalation exposure study was estimated to be below 1.5 mg/m^3.

4.3.3 *Simplified In Vitro Method for NCM Inhalation Toxicity Assessment*

Under the NEDO project (FY2017–2019), intratracheal instillation methods were established for three representative CNF types. However, as the range of NCM applications expands, it is increasingly impractical to evaluate all material types using animal studies due to their high cost and extended duration. Furthermore, in line with the 3Rs principle (Replacement, Reduction, and Refinement), there is growing international emphasis on the development of nonanimal alternative approaches, including in vitro cell-based assays, for safety evaluation.

Compared with animal studies, in vitro assays can be conducted more rapidly and in smaller-scale facilities and have been widely applied in toxicity assessments of various engineered nanomaterials. Our research group has previously reported multiple findings on this topic (Fujita et al. 2009, 2013, 2015a, 2018, 2020). Nevertheless, in vitro inhalation toxicity assessments of NCMs have not yet reached sufficient maturity at the international level.

Against this background, the NEDO project (FY2020–2024) aimed to develop and validate simple and rapid in vitro assessment methods for evaluating the inhalation toxicity of diverse NCMs. Although such assays cannot fully reproduce in vivo responses, they are expected to complement animal studies by providing mechanistic insights into cellular level reactions, thereby supporting comparative assessment and risk evaluation. An overview of the research framework is presented in Fig. 4.7.

4.3.3.1 Preparation and Characterization of NCMs for In Vitro Assays

Based on previous in vitro studies of engineered nanomaterials and the physicochemical properties of NCM suspensions, the NEDO project (FY2020–2024) identified four critical factors affecting the reliability of cellular assays for NCMs: (1) endotoxin contamination, (2) microbial contamination, (3) adsorption of culture medium components onto NCM surfaces, and (4) changes in agglomeration and

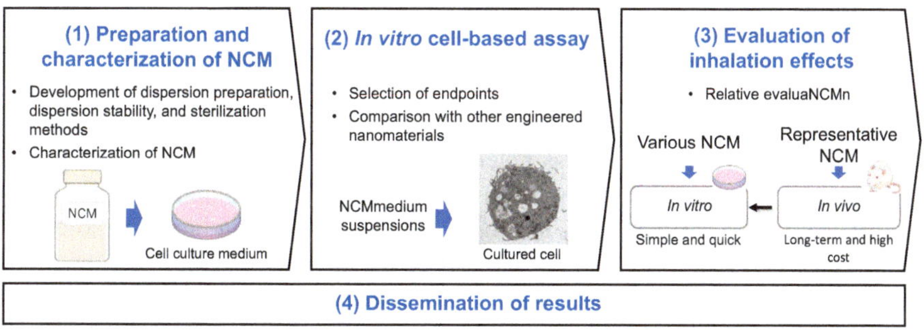

Fig. 4.7 Framework for the development of an assessment approach for the inhalation effects of NCMs

dispersion behavior resulting from interactions with culture medium constituents. To address these challenges, relevant literature was systematically reviewed, and a comprehensive article summarizing key issues and mitigation strategies for in vitro testing of NCMs was prepared and published (Moriyama et al. 2023).

Typical cell culture media contain salts, amino acids, sugars, trace nutrients, and additives such as fetal bovine serum (FBS), antibiotics, and antifungal agents. NCMs—particularly CNFs—exhibit distinctive properties such as thixotropy, promote agglomeration in these media and adsorption of serum proteins onto their surfaces. Consequently, optimization of sample preparation and rigorous physicochemical characterization are essential for ensuring reproducibility and reliability in cell-based assays. Recent studies have emphasized that dispersion preparation methods critically influence the validity of safety assessments for cellulose-based materials (Zhang et al. 2024).

In this study, preparation protocols were developed to obtain stable CNF dispersions, minimize agglomeration, and maintain biological safety. Comprehensive characterization was performed to assess both physicochemical and biological properties (Fig. 4.8). Particular attention was paid to microbial contamination and the presence of endotoxins, as plant-derived cellulose may serve as a substrate that supports the growth of bacteria and fungi. The results demonstrated that antibiotics, heat treatment, and autoclaving effectively eliminated microorganisms from CNF suspensions; however, heat treatment and autoclaving adversely affected the physicochemical integrity of CNFs and were ineffective in deactivating endotoxins and β-glucans (Fujita et al. 2023c). Accordingly, while antibiotics may suppress microbial growth in in vitro studies, the potential biological effects of residual endotoxins and β-glucans should also be taken into account when interpreting assay results.

As described in Sect. 4.3.1.1, gamma irradiation was adopted as a sterilization method that effectively inactivates microorganisms while preserving the physicochemical properties of CNFs. This approach enabled the establishment of a standardized sterilization protocol applicable to both in vitro and in vivo studies (Horie et al. 2023).

4.3.3.2 In Vitro Cell-Based Studies

4.3.3.2.1 Evaluation of CNF Effects Using Rat Alveolar Macrophages

Cytotoxicity and inflammatory responses to CNFs were evaluated using rat alveolar macrophages (NR8383) to assess potential pulmonary effects at the cellular level (Fujita et al. 2025c). Six CNF types were examined: TEMPO-oxidized CNFs, phosphorylated CNFs, mechanically fibrillated CNFs derived from bleached softwood kraft pulp, CNFs derived from citrus peels (Hideno et al. 2019), and coarse and ultrafine CNF fractions produced from bleached softwood kraft pulp using the aqueous counter collision (ACC) method (Kose et al. 2011).

No marked generation of ROS was observed in any CNF-exposed group. However, exposure to TEMPO-oxidized CNFs, phosphorylated CNFs, and

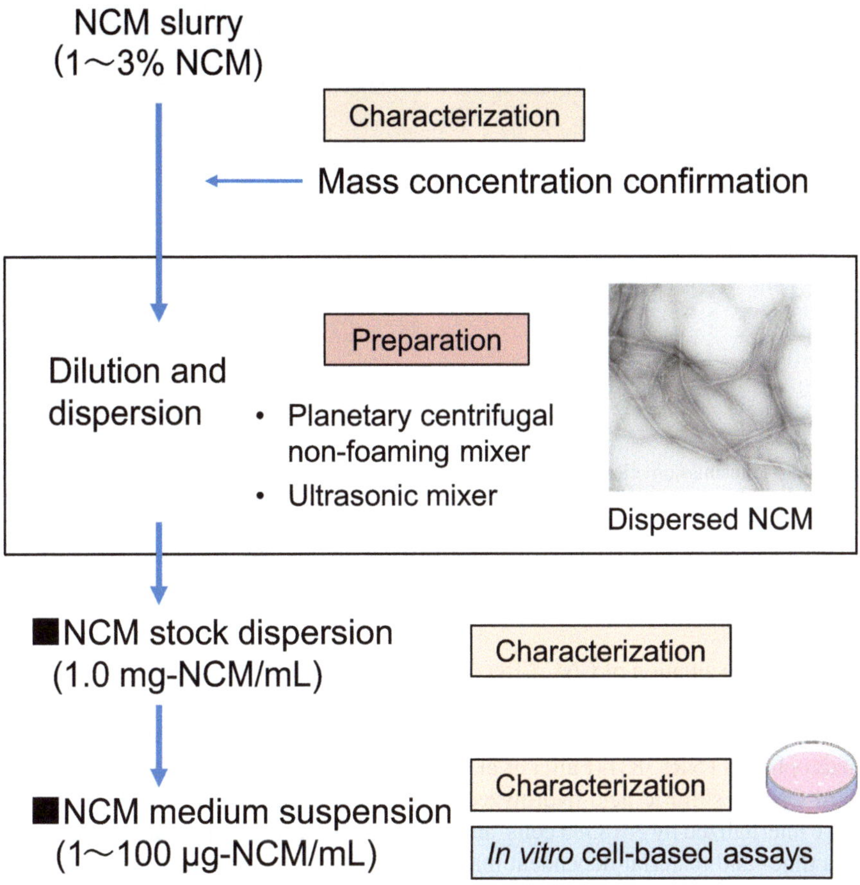

Fig. 4.8 Development of preparation methods and characterization protocols for NCM dispersions used in in vitro cell-based assays

mechanically fibrillated CNFs resulted in increased mitochondrial dehydrogenase activity, elevated production of proinflammatory cytokines, and induction of inflammation-related gene expression. In contrast, CNFs derived from citrus peels and both ACC-derived fractions showed no pronounced effects across these endpoints. Furthermore, no clear correlation was observed between biological contamination (e.g., bacteria or endotoxins) in CNF suspensions and cytotoxic responses, suggesting that CNFs themselves do not inherently exhibit significant cytotoxicity. A complementary study using fluorescently labeled CNFs confirmed phagocytosis by NR8383 cells within 24 h of exposure (Fig. 4.9).

These findings indicate that certain CNFs can induce moderate activation of alveolar macrophages, whereas others exhibit minimal biological activity. The results further suggest that the biological responses to CNFs are strongly influenced by factors such as raw material source, manufacturing process, and physicochemical characteristics, underscoring the importance of case-by-case safety evaluation.

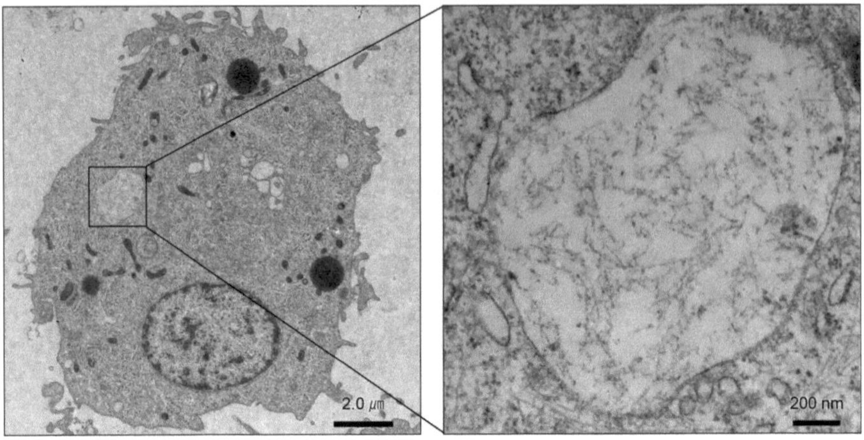

Fig. 4.9 Transmission electron micrographs showing phagocytosis of fluorescently labeled TEMPO-oxidized cellulose nanofibrils (CNFs) by NR8383 rat alveolar macrophages. The left panel shows an overview of a macrophage containing intracellular vesicular structures. The boxed region is enlarged in the right panel, revealing fibrous CNF structures within a membrane-bound intracellular compartment, indicating cellular uptake and retention of CNFs. Scale bars = 2.0 μm (*left*) and 200 nm (*right*)

4.3.3.2.2 Evaluation of CNC Effects Using Rat Alveolar Macrophages

The cytotoxic and immunological effects of CNCs were evaluated using rat alveolar macrophages (NR8383) (Fujita et al. 2025b). Three CNC types were tested: standard CNC1, sulfuric acid-hydrolyzed CNC2, and desulfurized CNC3. All CNCs were internalized by NR8383 cells, and inflammatory cytokine production increased in a time- and material-dependent manner. In particular, CNC2 and CNC3 induced marked increases in cytokines including IL-1α, IL-1β, IL-6, IL-18, MCP-1, MIP-1α, and TNFα, with CNC2 also significantly increasing GM-CSF levels. TEM confirmed cellular uptake, revealing electron-dense CNC1 particles localized within vacuole-like structures.

Cell viability assays showed no significant effects after 24 h of exposure; however, after 48 h, CNC3 (100 μg/mL) significantly reduced cell viability, indicating time-dependent cytotoxic effect. CNC1 and CNC2 exhibited only minor effects. Gene expression analysis revealed that CNC2 elicited the strongest transcriptional response, with significant upregulation of genes associated with inflammation, oxidative stress, apoptosis, and extracellular matrix degradation, including *Ccl5*, *Ccl12*, *Hmox1*, *Serpine1*, *Sod2*, *Mmp3*, *Mmp9*, and *Mmp12*.

Collectively, these findings demonstrate that CNCs can induce inflammatory responses in alveolar macrophages, with CNC2 and CNC3 producing pronounced cytokine release and transcriptional changes, and CNC3 exhibiting mild to moderate cytotoxicity upon prolonged exposure. Overall, the biological effects of CNCs appear to be strongly influenced by particle morphology and surface chemistry, underscoring the importance of physicochemical properties as key determinants of cellular responses.

4.3.3.2.3 Microbial Inactivation and Cellular Response Evaluation by Gamma Irradiation

Evaluation of microbial contamination in CNF suspensions and its influence on in vitro cell-based assays revealed the presence of microorganisms as well as LPS-like biological activity (Horie et al. 2023). To address these contaminants, gamma irradiation was applied at absorbed doses of 0.5, 1, 5, and 10 kGy, followed by assessment of the resulting cellular responses using six cultured cell types (HaCaT, A549, Caco-2, MeT-5A, THP-1, and NR8383). Irradiation at 1 kGy reduced microbial contamination and exerted bactericidal effects while preserving CNF physicochemical properties. In contrast, irradiation at 10 kGy achieved complete sterilization but shortened fiber length. CNF suspensions induced LPS-like cellular responses, particularly strong IL-8 induction in macrophage cell lines, and this activity persisted even after irradiation at doses of 10 kGy or higher. These findings indicate that while gamma irradiation is effective for microbial inactivation in CNF suspensions, it does not eliminate LPS-like biological activity. Consequently, such residual activity must be carefully considered when interpreting in vitro cytotoxicity results.

4.3.3.2.4 Evaluation Using a Three-Dimensional Human Airway Model

The cytotoxicity potential of CNFs was further evaluated using a three-dimensional (3D) human airway tissue model designed to mimic human respiratory epithelium. The tested materials included slurries of TEMPO-oxidized CNFs, phosphorylated CNFs, and mechanically fibrillated CNFs derived from softwood bleached kraft pulp. CNF stock solutions (1000 μg/mL) were prepared by mixing slurries with ultrapure water using a planetary centrifugal mixer and subsequently diluted with culture medium to a final concentration of 100 μg/mL. After culturing the 3D airway tissues, CNF dispersions were applied to the apical surface and incubated for 24 h. Cytotoxicity was assessed by measuring LDH release as an indicator of cell membrane damage. No significant cytotoxicity was observed for any CNF sample compared with vehicle controls. Although inflammatory responses were also evaluated, no marked changes were detected in the expression of inflammation-related genes under the experimental conditions tested (Moriyama et al. 2023). Taken together, these results suggest that CNFs do not exert acute cytotoxic effects in a physiologically relevant human airway tissue model under the conditions tested.

4.3.4 Dissemination of Research Outcomes

Under the NEDO project (FY2017–2019), a Japanese-language version of the *Testing Manual for the Toxicological Evaluation of Cellulose Nanofibers* was developed in 2020, based on standardized testing methods and case studies established during the project. In 2023, the English edition, *A Manual for Toxicity Testing of*

Cellulose Nanofibers, was published (Fujita et al. 2023a). During the subsequent NEDO project (FY2020–2024), comprehensive safety evaluation reports on NCMs were published in 2022 and 2025, providing detailed assessments of inhalation, dermal, and oral exposure routes.

These documents are freely available through the website of the Research Institute for Science and Safety, AIST, and through the Nano Safety Website operated by the same institute. (https://riss.aist.go.jp/) and on the Nano Safety Website operated by the same institute (https://riss.aist.go.jp/nanosafety/).

In addition, the project outcomes were disseminated through a series of peer-reviewed publications. Major contributions include:

- Reviews on the inhalation effects of CNFs (Sai and Fujita 2020; Fujita 2024; Fujita and Moriyama 2025)
- Studies on sterilization methods for CNF suspensions (Sai et al. 2020)
- Studies using intratracheal instillation of NCMs (Fujita et al. 2021, 2023b, 2025a, 2025b; Yamashita et al. 2024)
- Reports on inhalation exposure studies of CNFs (Yamashita et al. 2025)
- A review addressing challenges in in vitro CNF testing (Moriyama et al. 2023)
- Studies on cellular responses to CNFs (Horie et al. 2023; Fujita et al. 2025c)
- Studies on cellular responses to CNCs (Fujita et al. 2025b)

Through these efforts, scientific knowledge and standardized methodologies for the safety assessment of NCMs have been made publicly available, establishing a foundational evidence base for future risk assessment and international standardization. These outputs support regulatory decision-making and provide essential scientific guidance for the safe and sustainable application of NCMs in industrial and biomedical fields.

4.4 Summary

Integrated Discussion

The existing literature generally indicates that short-term exposure to NCMs, including CNFs and CNCs, induces transient pulmonary inflammatory responses comparable to those observed for conventional cellulose and other poorly soluble, low-toxicity dusts. These effects differ markedly from the more severe pulmonary outcomes reported for certain high-rigidity, long, and biopersistent CNTs (e.g., specific MWCNT types) and for asbestos. CNTs are not a monolithic class; pulmonary hazard varies with morphology, rigidity, surface chemistry, and biopersistence. Inhalation studies further suggest that CNFs tend to elicit milder inflammatory responses than CNCs. Overall, both CNFs and CNCs appear less likely than these high-hazard CNT exemplars to induce serious pulmonary outcomes such as sustained inflammation, fibrosis, granuloma formation, or epithelial hyperplasia, largely due to differences in rigidity, morphology, surface chemistry, and biopersistence. Nevertheless, uncertainties remain regarding NCM persistence in lung tissue and potential chronic effects following uptake.

The NEDO projects (FY2017–2019 and FY2020–2024) provided insights that extend beyond prior studies. Chemically modified CNFs with smaller fiber diameters induced alveolar inflammation that resolved within 90 days, whereas mechanically fibrillated CNFs with larger diameters produced milder responses and preferentially accumulated around terminal bronchioles as well as alveoli. Compared with MWCNTs, all tested NCMs exhibited markedly lower inflammatory potential. Phagocytosis by alveolar macrophages persisted even after resolution of inflammation, indicating continued cellular retention despite the absence of overt inflammatory responses. CNFs demonstrated slow clearance and long-term retention, with deposition patterns influenced by fiber diameter and length. Importantly, no evidence of systemic immunotoxicity was observed following short-term exposure.

Collectively, these findings emphasize the necessity of evaluating NCMs on an individual basis according to their physicochemical characteristics rather than treating them as a homogeneous material class. They also underscore the importance of integrating in vivo and in vitro data to establish a robust, science-based risk assessment framework that reflects realistic exposure scenarios.

Key Points from Literature

- Short-term NCM exposure generally induces transient pulmonary inflammation, distinct from the more severe effects reported for asbestos and for certain long, rigid, and biopersistent CNTs.
- CNFs typically elicit milder inflammation than CNCs.
- Compared with high-rigidity, long, and biopersistent CNT types, NCMs appear less likely to cause fibrosis, granulomas, or tumorigenesis under comparable experimental conditions.
- Long-term persistence and clearance kinetics remain insufficiently understood.

Key Findings from NEDO Projects

- Chemically modified CNFs induced alveolar inflammation that resolved within 90 days.
- Mechanically fibrillated CNFs elicited milder pulmonary responses and predominantly accumulated near terminal bronchioles.
- NCMs exhibited significantly lower inflammatory potential than MWCNTs.
- Persistent macrophage phagocytosis and slow clearance suggest long-term pulmonary retention.
- No systemic immunotoxicity was observed after short-term exposure.

Future Challenges

- Long-term studies to clarify chronic effects and clearance kinetics.
- Evaluation of immune modulation beyond local pulmonary inflammation, including potential systemic effects following long-term exposure.
- Alignment of experimental exposure scenarios with real-world conditions through inhalation studies using aerosolized NCMs.

- Systematic analysis of physicochemical factors, including fiber dimensions, aspect ratio, morphology, and surface chemistry, that influence toxicity.
- Improved in vitro models addressing dispersion stability, endotoxin control, and multiendpoint biomarkers.

  Development of integrated risk assessment frameworks combining in vivo and in vitro data to support regulatory decision-making.

References

Adamis Z, Tátrai E, Honma K, Ungváry G (1997) *In vitro* and *in vivo* assessment of the pulmonary toxicity of cellulose. J Appl Toxicol 17(2):137–141. https://doi.org/10.1002/(SICI)1099-1263(199703)17:2<137::AID-JAT423>3.0.CO;2-I

Aimonen K, Imani M, Hartikainen M, Suhonen S, Vanhala E, Moreno C, Rojas OJ, Norppa H, Catalán J (2022) Surface functionalization and size modulate the formation of reactive oxygen species and genotoxic effects of cellulose nanofibrils. Part Fibre Toxicol 19(1):19. https://doi.org/10.1186/s12989-022-00460-3

Bhattacharya K, Kiliç G, Costa PM, Fadeel B (2017) Cytotoxicity screening and cytokine profiling of nineteen nanomaterials enables hazard ranking and grouping based on inflammogenic potential. Nanotoxicology 11(6):809–826. https://doi.org/10.1080/17435390.2017.1363309

Catalán J, Rydman E, Aimonen K, Hannukainen KS, Suhonen S, Vanhala E, Moreno C, Meyer V, Perez DD, Sneck A, Forsström U, Højgaard C, Willemoes M, Winther JR, Vogel U, Wolff H, Alenius H, Savolainen KM, Norppa H (2017) Genotoxic and inflammatory effects of nanofibrillated cellulose in murine lungs. Mutagenesis 32(1):23–31. https://doi.org/10.1093/mutage/gew035

Čolić M, Tomić S, Bekić M (2020) Immunological aspects of nanocellulose. Immunol Lett 222:80–89. https://doi.org/10.1016/j.imlet.2020.04.004

Ede JD, Ong KJ, Goergen M, Rudie A, Pomeroy-Carter CA, Shatkin JA (2019) Risk analysis of cellulose nanomaterials by inhalation: current state of science. Nanomaterials (Basel) 9(3):337. https://doi.org/10.3390/nano9030337

Farcas MT, Kisin ER, Menas AL, Gutkin DW, Star A, Reiner RS, Yanamala N, Savolainen K, Shvedova AA (2016) Pulmonary exposure to cellulose nanocrystals caused deleterious effects to reproductive system in male mice. J Toxicol Environ Health A 79(21):984–997. https://doi.org/10.1080/15287394.2016.1211045

Fujita K (2024) Assessing inhalation toxicity of cellulose nanofibrils. Oleoscience 24(5):197–203. (in Japanese). https://doi.org/10.5650/oleoscience.24.197

Fujita K, Moriyama A (2025) Inhalation toxicity of cellulose nanofibrils: a review of key findings and future directions. Carbohydr Polym Technol Appl 11:100913. https://doi.org/10.1016/j.carpta.2025.100913

Fujita K, Horie M, Kato H, Endoh S, Suzuki M, Nakamura A, Miyauchi A, Yamamoto K, Kinugasa S, Nishio K, Yoshida Y, Iwahashi H, Nakanishi J (2009) Effects of ultrafine TiO2 particles on gene expression profile in human keratinocytes without illumination: involvement of extracellular matrix and cell adhesion. Toxicol Lett 191(2–3):109–117. https://doi.org/10.1016/j.toxlet.2009.08.011

Fujita K, Morimoto Y, Ogami A, Myojyo T, Tanaka I, Shimada M, Wang WN, Endoh S, Uchida K, Nakazato T, Yamamoto K, Fukui H, Horie M, Yoshida Y, Iwahashi H, Nakanishi J (2009a) Gene expression profiles in rat lung after inhalation exposure to C60 fullerene particles$_{60}$ fullerene particles. Toxicology 258(1):47–55. https://doi.org/10.1016/j.tox.2009.01.005

Fujita K, Morimoto Y, Ogami A, Tanaka I, Endoh S, Uchida K, Tao H, Akasaka M, Inada M, Yamamoto K, Fukui H, Hayakawa M, Horie M, Saito Y, Yoshida Y, Iwahashi H, Niki E,

Nakanishi J (2009b) A gene expression profiling approach to study the influence of ultrafine particles on rat lungs. In: Kim YJ, Platt U, Gu MB, Iwahashi H (eds) Atmospheric and biological environmental monitoring. Springer Netherlands, pp 219–227. https://doi.org/10.1007/978-1-4020-9674-7_14

Fujita K, Morimoto Y, Endoh S, Uchida K, Fukui H, Ogami A, Tanaka I, Horie M, Yoshida Y, Iwahashi H, Nakanishi J (2010) Identification of potential biomarkers from gene expression profiles in rat lungs intratracheally instilled with C(60) fullerenes$_{60}$ fullerenes. Toxicology 274(1–3):34–41. https://doi.org/10.1016/j.tox.2010.05.004

Fujita K, Fukuda M, Endoh S, Kato H, Maru J, Nakamura A, Uchino K, Shinohara N, Obara S, Nagano R, Horie M, Kinugasa S, Hashimoto H, Kishimoto A (2013) Physical properties of single-wall carbon nanotubes in cell culture and their dispersal due to alveolar epithelial cell response. Toxicol Mech Methods 23(8):598–609. https://doi.org/10.3109/15376516.2013.811568

Fujita K, Fukuda M, Endoh S, Maru J, Kato H, Nakamura A, Shinohara N, Uchino K, Honda K (2015a) Size effects of single-walled carbon nanotubes on *in vivo* and *in vitro* pulmonary toxicity. Inhal Toxicol 27(4):207–223. https://doi.org/10.3109/08958378.2015.1026620

Fujita K, Fukuda M, Fukui H, Horie M, Endoh S, Uchida K, Shichiri M, Morimoto Y, Ogami A, Iwahashi H (2015b) Intratracheal instillation of single-wall carbon nanotubes in the rat lung induces time-dependent changes in gene expression. Nanotoxicology 9(3):290–301. https://doi.org/10.3109/17435390.2014.921737

Fujita K, Fukuda M, Endoh S, Maru J, Kato H, Nakamura A, Shinohara N, Uchino K, Honda K (2016) Pulmonary and pleural inflammation after intratracheal instillation of short single-walled and multi-walled carbon nanotubes. Toxicol Lett 257:23–37. https://doi.org/10.1016/j.toxlet.2016.05.025

Fujita K, Take S, Tani R, Maru J, Obara S, Endoh S (2018) Assessment of cytotoxicity and mutagenicity of exfoliated graphene. Toxicol in Vitro 52:195–202. https://doi.org/10.1016/j.tiv.2018.06.016

Fujita K, Obara S, Maru J, Endoh S (2020) Cytotoxicity profiles of multi-walled carbon nanotubes with different physico-chemical properties. Toxicol Mech Methods 30(7):477–489. https://doi.org/10.1080/15376516.2020.1761920

Fujita K, Obara S, Maru J, Endoh S (2021) Pulmonary inflammation following intratracheal instillation of cellulose nanofibrils in rats: comparison with multi-walled carbon nanotubes. Cellulose 28(11):7143–7164. https://doi.org/10.1007/s10570-021-03943-2

Fujita K, Endoh S, Maru J, Sai T, Tomoko A, Goi Y, Obara S, Tani F, Yamamoto F, Ogawa T (2023a) A manual for toxicity testing of cellulose nanofibers. https://riss.aist.go.jp/results-and-dissemin/776/

Fujita K, Obara S, Maru J, Endoh S (2023b) Effects of advanced nanomaterials on the respiratory system of a murine COPD model. Toxicol Rep 11:481–492. https://doi.org/10.1016/j.toxrep.2023.11.009

Fujita K, Obara S, Maru J, Endoh S, Moriyama A, Horie M (2023c) Biological characterization of cellulose nanofibril suspensions. J Toxicol Sci (50th Annual Meeting of the Japanese Society of Toxicology) 48(Suppl):2–155

Fujita K, Obara S, Maru J, Kawai Y, Endoh S (2025a) Pulmonary inflammatory responses and retention dynamics of cellulose nanofibrils. Toxicology 511:154038. https://doi.org/10.1016/j.tox.2024.154038

Fujita K, Obara S, Maru J, Kawai Y, Endoh S, Moriyama A (2025b) Pulmonary inflammation and immune responses induced by nanocellulose: insights from *in vivo* and *in vitro* models. Curr Res Toxicol 9:100259. https://doi.org/10.1016/j.crtox.2025.100259

Fujita K, Obara S, Maru J, Endoh S, Kawai Y, Moriyama A, Horie M (2025c) Assessing cytotoxicity and biocompatibility of cellulose nanofibrils on alveolar macrophages. Cellulose 32(1):241–260. https://doi.org/10.1007/s10570-024-06238-4

Hadrup N, Knudsen KB, Berthing T, Wolff H, Bengtson S, Kofoed C, Espersen R, Højgaard C, Winther JR, Willemoës M, Wedin I, Nuopponen M, Alenius H, Norppa H, Wallin H, Vogel

U (2019) Pulmonary effects of nanofibrillated celluloses in mice suggest that carboxylation lowers the inflammatory and acute phase responses. Environ Toxicol Pharmacol 66:116–125. https://doi.org/10.1016/j.etap.2019.01.003

Hideno A, Abe K, Yano H, Uchimura H (2019) Characterization of nanofibers from Japanese orange inner peels prepared using pectinase and diluted alkali. J Jpn Inst Energy 98(5):85–89. https://doi.org/10.3775/jie.98.85

Honda K, Naya M, Takehara H, Kataura H, Fujita K, Ema M (2017) A 104-week pulmonary toxicity assessment of long and short single-wall carbon nanotubes after a single intratracheal instillation in rats. Inhal Toxicol 29(11):471–482. https://doi.org/10.1080/08958378.2017.1394930

Horie M, Fujita K, Endoh S, Sugino S, Maru J, Moriyama A, Ogura I (2023) Contaminant microorganisms in the *in vitro* evaluation of cellular responses of cellulose nanofibers and their microbial inactivation using gamma irradiation. Toxicol Mech Methods 33(9):741–754. https://doi.org/10.1080/15376516.2023.2238061

Ilves M, Vilske S, Aimonen K, Lindberg HK, Pesonen S, Wedin I, Nuopponen M, Vanhala E, Højgaard C, Winther JR, Willemoës M, Vogel U, Wolff H, Norppa H, Savolainen K, Alenius H (2018) Nanofibrillated cellulose causes acute pulmonary inflammation that subsides within a month. Nanotoxicology 12(7):729–746. https://doi.org/10.1080/17435390.2018.1472312

ISO (1995) ISO 7708:1995, air quality—particle size fraction definitions for health-related sampling

Joseph P, Umbright CM, Roberts JR, Cumpston JL, Orandle MS, McKinney WG, Sager TM (2021) Lung toxicity and gene expression changes in response to whole-body inhalation exposure to cellulose nanocrystal in rats. Inhal Toxicol 33(2):66–80. https://doi.org/10.1080/08958378.2021.1884320

Kasai T, Umeda Y, Ohnishi M, Mine T, Kondo H, Takeuchi T, Matsumoto M, Fukushima S (2016) Lung carcinogenicity of inhaled multi-walled carbon nanotube in rats. Part Fibre Toxicol 13(1):53. https://doi.org/10.1186/s12989-016-0164-2

Kose R, Mitani I, Kasai W, Kondo T (2011) 'Nanocellulose' as a single nanofiber prepared from pellicle secreted by *Gluconacetobacter xylinus* using aqueous counter collision. Biomacromolecules 12(3):716–720. https://doi.org/10.1021/bm1013469

Lopes VR, Sanchez-Martinez C, Strømme M, Ferraz N (2017) *In vitro* biological responses to nanofibrillated cellulose by human dermal, lung and immune cells: surface chemistry aspect. Part Fibre Toxicol 14(1):1. https://doi.org/10.1186/s12989-016-0182-0

Menas AL, Yanamala N, Farcas MT, Russo M, Friend S, Fournier PM, Star A, Iavicoli I, Shurin GV, Vogel UB, Fadeel B, Beezhold D, Kisin ER, Shvedova AA (2017) Fibrillar vs crystalline nanocellulose pulmonary epithelial cell responses: cytotoxicity or inflammation? Chemosphere 171:671–680. https://doi.org/10.1016/j.chemosphere.2016.12.105

Mercer RR, Hubbs AF, Scabilloni JF, Wang L, Battelli LA, Friend S, Castranova V, Porter DW (2011) Pulmonary fibrotic response to aspiration of multi-walled carbon nanotubes. Part Fibre Toxicol 8:21. https://doi.org/10.1186/1743-8977-8-21

Milton DK, Godleski JJ, Feldman HA, Greaves IA (1990) Toxicity of intratracheally instilled cotton dust, cellulose, and endotoxin. Am Rev Respir Dis 142(1):184–192. https://doi.org/10.1164/ajrccm/142.1.184

Moriyama A, Ogura I, Fujita K (2023) Potential issues specific to cytotoxicity tests of cellulose nanofibrils. J Appl Toxicol 43(1):195–207. https://doi.org/10.1002/jat.4390

Murphy FA, Poland CA, Duffin R, Al-Jamal KT, Ali-Boucetta H, Nunes A, Byrne F, Prina-Mello A, Volkov Y, Li S, et al. (2011) Length-dependent retention of carbon nanotubes in the pleural space of mice initiates sustained inflammation and progressive fibrosis on the parietal pleura. American Journal of Pathology 178(6):2587–2600. https://doi.org/10.1016/j.ajpath.2011.02.040

Nagato LK, Lourenço MG, Cadete RA, Leite-Júnior JH, Koatz VL, Rocco PR, Faffe DS, Zin WA (2008) Microcrystalline cellulose induces time-dependent lung functional and inflammatory changes. Respir Physiol Neurobiol 164(3):331–337. https://doi.org/10.1016/j.resp.2008.08.005

OECD (2018a) Test no. 412: subacute inhalation toxicity: 28-day study, OECD guidelines for the testing of chemicals, section 4. OECD Publishing, Paris. https://doi.org/10.1787/9789264070783-en

OECD (2018b) Test no. 413: subchronic inhalation toxicity: 90-day study, OECD guidelines for the testing of chemicals, section 4. OECD Publishing, Paris. https://doi.org/10.1787/9789264070806-en

OECD (2024) Test no. 403: acute inhalation toxicity, OECD guidelines for the testing of chemicals, section 4. OECD Publishing, Paris. https://doi.org/10.1787/9789264070608-en

Ogura I, Kajihara H, Kuboyama T, Oguri T, Kawamoto A, Gamo M (2020) Examples of emission and exposure assessment of cellulose nanofibers and their applied products (in Japanese). https://riss.aist.go.jp/results-and-dissemin/776/

Ogura I, Moriyama A, Iizumi Y, Endoh S, Fujita K, Horie M, Okazaki T, Matsuzawa T (2025) Effect of gamma irradiation on cellulose nanofibers. J Wood Sci 71(1):37. https://doi.org/10.1186/s10086-025-02215-y

Park EJ, Khaliullin TO, Shurin MR, Kisin ER, Yanamala N, Fadeel B, Chang J, Shvedova AA (2018) Fibrous nanocellulose, crystalline nanocellulose, carbon nanotubes, and crocidolite asbestos elicit disparate immune responses upon pharyngeal aspiration in mice. J Immunotoxicol 15(1):12–23. https://doi.org/10.1080/1547691X.2017.1414339

Pinto F, Lourenço AF, Pedrosa JFS, Gonçalves L, Ventura C, Vital N, Bettencourt A, Fernandes SN, da Rosa RR, Godinho MH, Louro H, Ferreira PJT, Silva MJ (2022) Analysis of the *in vitro* toxicity of nanocelluloses in human lung cells as compared to multi-walled carbon nanotubes. Nanomaterials (Basel) 12(9):1432. https://doi.org/10.3390/nano12091432

Porter DW, Hubbs AF, Mercer RR, Wu N, Wolfarth MG, Sriram K, Leonard S, Battelli L, Schwegler-Berry D, Friend S, Andrew M, Chen BT, Tsuruoka S, Endo M, Castranova V (2010) Mouse pulmonary dose- and time course-responses induced by exposure to multi-walled carbon nanotubes. Toxicology 269(2–3):136–147. https://doi.org/10.1016/j.tox.2009.10.017

Sai T, Fujita K (2020) A review of pulmonary toxicity studies of nanocellulose. Inhal Toxicol 32(6):231–239. https://doi.org/10.1080/08958378.2020.1770901

Sai T, Maru J, Obara S, Endoh S, Kajihara H, Fujita K (2020) Screening of preservatives and evaluation of sterilized cellulose nanofibers for toxicity studies. J Occup Health 62(1):e12176. https://doi.org/10.1002/1348-9585.12176

Shatkin JA, Ong KJ, Ede JD, Wegner TH, Goergen M (2016) Toward cellulose nanomaterial commercialization: knowledge gap analysis for Safety Data Sheets according to the Globally Harmonized System. TAPPI J 15(6):425–437. https://doi.org/10.32964/TJ15.6.425

Shvedova AA, Kisin ER, Yanamala N, Farcas MT, Menas AL, Williams A, Fournier PM, Reynolds JS, Gutkin DW, Star A, Reiner RS, Halappanavar S, Kagan VE (2016) Gender differences in murine pulmonary responses elicited by cellulose nanocrystals. Part Fibre Toxicol 13(1):28. https://doi.org/10.1186/s12989-016-0140-x

Song LY, Wu YZ, Pei XX, Li R, Chen HT, Sun XZ (2020) Pulmonary toxicity and RNA sequencing analyses of mouse in response to exposure to cellulose nanofibrils. Inhal Toxicol 32(9–10):388–401. https://doi.org/10.1080/08958378.2020.1831112

Stoudmann N, Schmutz M, Hirsch C, Nowack B, Som C (2020) Human hazard potential of nanocellulose: quantitative insights from the literature. Nanotoxicology 14(9):1241–1257. https://doi.org/10.1080/17435390.2020.1814440

Tátrai E, Adamis Z, Böhm U, Merétey K, Ungváry G (1995) Role of cellulose in wood dust-induced fibrosing alveo-bronchiolitis in rat. J Appl Toxicol 15(1):45–48. https://doi.org/10.1002/jat.2550150110

Tátrai E, Brozik M, Adamis Z, Merétey K, Ungváry G (1996) *In vivo* pulmonary toxicity of cellulose in rats. J Appl Toxicol 16(2):129–135. https://doi.org/10.1002/(SICI)1099-1263(199603)16:2<129::AID-JAT316>3.0.CO;2-C

Ventura C, Pinto F, Lourenço AF, Ferreira PJT, Louro H, Silva MJ (2020) On the toxicity of cellulose nanocrystals and nanofibrils in animal and cellular models. Cellulose 27(10):5509–5544. https://doi.org/10.1007/s10570-020-03176-9

Yamashita Y, Tokunaga A, Aoki K, Ishizuka T, Uematsu H, Sakamoto H, Fujita S, Tanoue S (2024) Assessing the safety of mechanically fibrillated cellulose nanofibers (fib-CNF) via toxicity tests on mice: single intratracheal administration and 28 days' oral intake. Toxics 12(2):121. https://doi.org/10.3390/toxics12020121

Yamashita Y, Tokunaga A, Aoki K, Ishizuka T, Fujita S, Tanoue S (2025) Safety of mechanically fibrillated cellulose nanofibers (CNFs) by inhalation exposure based on TG412. Nanomaterials (Basel) 15(3):214. https://doi.org/10.3390/nano15030214

Yamato H (1994) Biological effects of inhaled fibrous particles. Earozoru Kenkyu 9(3):215–220. (in Japanese)

Yanamala N, Farcas MT, Hatfield MK, Kisin ER, Kagan VE, Geraci CL, Shvedova AA (2014) *In vivo* evaluation of the pulmonary toxicity of cellulose nanocrystals: a renewable and sustainable nanomaterial of the future. ACS Sustain Chem Eng 2(7):1691–1698. https://doi.org/10.1021/sc500153k

Yanamala N, Kisin ER, Menas AL, Farcas MT, Khaliullin TO, Vogel UB, Shurin GV, Schwegler-Berry D, Fournier PM, Star A, Shvedova AA (2016) *In vitro* toxicity evaluation of lignin-(un) coated cellulose based nanomaterials on human A549 and THP-1 cells. Biomacromolecules 17(11):3464–3473. https://doi.org/10.1021/acs.biomac.6b00756

Zhang Y, Fox DM, Ong KJ, Ede J, Sayes C, Kangas H, Ilona L, Goergen M, Moon R, Shatkin JA (2024) Limitations of recent cellulose studies: how overzealous dispersion technique, fluorescence labeling and interpretation limit the findings of recent safety assessments for cellulose materials. Trends Food Sci Technol 151:104620. https://doi.org/10.1016/j.tifs.2024.104620

Chapter 5
Dermal Effects: Skin Barrier Interactions and Irritation Potential

Katsuhide Fujita

Abstract Dermal exposure is an important consideration in the safety evaluation of nanocellulose materials (NCMs), including cellulose nanofibrils (CNFs, also referred to as cellulose nanofibers) and cellulose nanocrystals (CNCs), as their use expands across consumer, industrial, and biomedical applications. This chapter provides an integrated assessment of skin permeation and barrier interactions, cytocompatibility, and irritation potential, synthesizing evidence from the published literature with findings from studies commissioned by the New Energy and Industrial Technology Development Organization (NEDO). Studies using cultured skin cells and reconstructed human epidermis models consistently show that CNFs and CNCs exhibit low cytotoxicity under typical exposure conditions and do not induce skin irritation when evaluated in accordance with OECD Test Guideline (TG) 439. Although surface chemistry, material form, and other material-specific factors may influence cellular responses, no significant adverse dermal effects have been reported. NEDO studies using 3D cultured human skin models demonstrated that TEMPO-oxidized CNFs remained confined to the outermost skin layers, with no detectable penetration into deeper tissues or receptor fluid. Overall, current evidence suggests a low potential for adverse dermal effects under realistic dermal exposure scenarios, while highlighting the importance of material-specific evaluation for prolonged skin contact.

Keywords Nanocellulose materials (NCMs) · Cellulose nanofibrils (CNFs) · Dermal exposure · Skin permeation · Skin irritation · 3D cultured human skin model · OECD Test Guideline 439

K. Fujita (✉)
Research Institute of Science for Safety and Sustainability (RISS), National Institute of Advanced Industrial Science and Technology (AIST), Tsukuba, Ibaraki, Japan
e-mail: ka-fujita@aist.go.jp

I. Ogura, K. Fujita (eds.), *Nanocellulose Materials*,
https://doi.org/10.1007/978-981-92-2148-6_5

5.1 Introduction

Nanocellulose materials (NCMs), including cellulose nanofibrils (CNFs, also referred to as cellulose nanofibers) and cellulose nanocrystals (CNCs), have expanded from their traditional applications in paper products and resin reinforcement into diverse sectors such as housing, agriculture, medical devices, and cosmetics. Their low density, high mechanical strength, and biodegradability have driven their adoption across a broad range of applications. As their use increases, opportunities for dermal exposure are expected to rise, raising concerns regarding occupational contact during manufacturing and processing, as well as potential risks associated with consumer use in daily life. The skin serves as the body's primary barrier against external agents and therefore plays a critical role in safety assessment. Key questions in the evaluation of dermal safety include whether nanostructured materials such as NCMs can penetrate the stratum corneum, undergo systemic absorption, or induce irritation and inflammatory responses. This chapter reviews current knowledge on the dermal effects of NCMs and discusses findings from skin permeation and irritation studies conducted under the New Energy and Industrial Technology Development Organization (NEDO) project (FY2017–2019), as well as remaining challenges for future research.

5.2 Information from Existing Literature

Evaluations of the dermal effects of CNFs and CNCs have primarily relied on in vitro assays using cultured skin cells and reconstructed skin models, reflecting the limited availability of in vivo and human data.

Kim et al. (2019) assessed CNFs intended for cosmetic applications by conducting cytotoxicity tests on HaCaT (immortalized human keratinocyte) cells and HDF-α fibroblasts, as well as skin and eye irritation tests using three-dimensional (3D) cultured models. Cytotoxicity was observed in a concentration-dependent manner, with effects noted at concentrations ≥156 μg/mL for HaCaT cells and ≥313 μg/mL for HDF-α cells. However, no clear irritation was detected in the 3D skin or eye models, highlighting the importance of appropriate concentration selection in dermal safety evaluation for cosmetic applications.

Lopes et al. (2017) compared the biological responses of unmodified and chemically modified nanofibrillated cellulose (NFC) gels, including carboxymethylated and cationically functionalized variants, using human dermal fibroblasts. None of the NFC gels induced cytotoxicity; moreover, although surface modifications may influence biological interactions, no significant adverse effects on cell viability or morphology were observed.

Nordli et al. (2016) investigated the cytotoxicity and metabolic activity of high-purity TEMPO-oxidized CNFs (endotoxin content: 45 EU/g) in human dermal fibroblasts and epidermal keratinocytes. CNF dispersions at 50 μg/mL showed no cytotoxicity and did not induce any of the 27 cytokines tested. While CNF aerogels slightly reduced cellular metabolic activity, they did not cause cell death and exhibited high moisture retention, suggesting potential suitability for wound dressing applications. These findings indicate that the dermal biological responses to CNFs may depend on both material form and exposure conditions.

Hua et al. (2014) examined the influence of nanostructure and surface modification on the biocompatibility of cellulose-based films. Using modified microfibrillated cellulose (MFC) and *Cladophora*-derived nanocellulose (CC; cellulose extracted from *Cladophora* algae) films, both indirect and direct contact assays confirmed the absence of toxic leachates and demonstrated noncytotoxic behavior. Carboxymethylated MFC and TEMPO-treated CC films exhibited particularly favorable biocompatibility, supporting cell adhesion and viability.

Ong et al. (2017) evaluated the skin irritation potential of BioPlus® lignin-coated CNFs (L-CNF) and CNCs (L-CNC) in accordance with Organisation for Economic Co-operation and Development (OECD) test guideline (TG) 439. Using the EpiDerm™ reconstructed human epidermis model with a 24-h exposure, both materials were classified as nonirritants under the globally harmonized system (GHS), indicating a low skin irritation potential under internationally harmonized regulatory criteria (Table 5.1).

5.3 Results of the NEDO Project

To comprehensively evaluate dermal safety, the NEDO project conducted studies on both skin permeation and irritation potential, which are summarized separately below. As the use of NCMs continues to expand across a wide range of products, opportunities for direct skin contact are expected to increase, underscoring the importance of these evaluations.

5.3.1 Skin Permeation Test

Evaluation of skin permeation is a critical component of dermal risk assessment. Traditionally, permeation tests have relied on excised skin from rats or pigs; however, increasing regulatory and ethical constraints—particularly in the EU—have accelerated the adoption of 3D cultured human skin models for regulatory safety assessments. These models, derived from human cells, reduce uncertainties associated with interspecies extrapolation and offer improved reproducibility, enabling reliable data generation for dermal safety evaluation.

In the NEDO project, a 3D cultured human skin model was employed to establish an evaluation method for CNF permeation (Fig. 5.1). Because accurate detection of trace amounts of CNFs within the skin model or receptor fluid was essential, specialized sample preparation and analytical techniques were developed to enable

Table 5.1 Summary of cell-based and reconstructed skin model studies evaluating the dermal effects of CNFs and CNCs

ID	Test material	Cell type	Exposure duration	Exposure concentration	Endpoints	References
1	CNFs	HaCaT, HDF-α, LabCyte EPI-MODEL24	24 h (HaCaT, HDF-α), 15 min (EPI-MODEL24)	≥156 μg/mL (HaCaT), ≥313 μg/mL (HDF-α), 1 wt% (EPI-MODEL24)	Cell viability/cytotoxicity, Skin irritation (OECD TG 439)	Kim et al. (2019)
2	Unmodified/modified NFCs	HDF, MRC-5 fibroblasts, THP-1 monocytes	24 h	50–500 μg/mL	Cytokine production, ROS generation, cell morphology	Lopes et al. (2017)
3	TEMPO-oxidized CNFs	Skin fibroblasts, keratinocytes	24 h	50 μg/mL	Cytotoxicity, cytokine production, cell morphology	Nordli et al. (2016)
4	Modified MFC and *Cladophora*-derived nanocellulose (CC)	HDF	24, 48 h	Not specified	Cytotoxicity, cell morphology	Hua et al. (2014)
5	Lignin-coated CNFs (L-CNF), Lignin-coated CNCs (L-CNC)	MatTek EpiDerm™	24 h	30–70 mg/mL	Skin irritation (OECD TG 439)	Ong et al. (2017)

Abbreviations: *HaCaT* immortalized human keratinocyte cell line, *HDF* human dermal fibroblasts, *NFC* nanofibrillated cellulose, *CNF* cellulose nanofibrils (also referred to as cellulose nanofibers), *CNC* cellulose nanocrystals

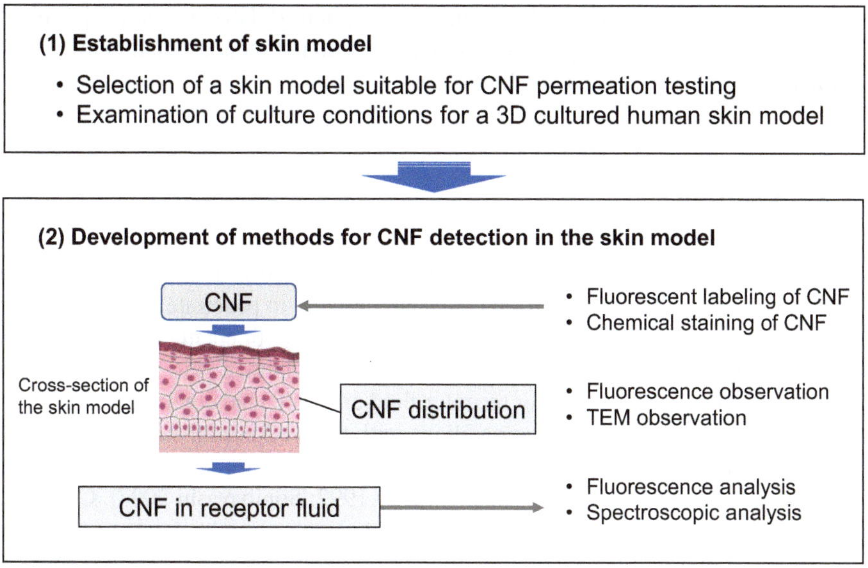

Fig. 5.1 Schematic illustration of the experimental framework for dermal permeation assessment and CNF detection using a 3D cultured human skin model

sensitive detection of CNFs. TEMPO-oxidized CNFs were selected as the test material, and two complementary visualization and detection strategies were implemented: chemical staining and fluorescent labeling through functional group modification. Methodological details are provided in *A Manual for Toxicity Testing of Cellulose Nanofibers* (Fujita et al. 2023a).

Permeation studies were conducted using static Franz diffusion cells equipped with the skin model. Chemically stained CNFs were not detected within the skin layers, and fluorescently labeled CNFs were not detected in the receptor fluid. In all cases, CNFs remained confined to the outermost surface layer of the skin model. These findings indicate that TEMPO-oxidized CNFs do not permeate the skin model and are unlikely to undergo percutaneous absorption under the tested experimental conditions.

5.3.2 Skin Irritation Test

The skin irritation potential of NCMs was evaluated in accordance with OECD TG 439 (OECD 2025). CNF dispersions were tested using two commercially available 3D cultured human skin models, EpiDerm™ EPI-200-SIT and SkinEthic™ RHE. TEMPO-oxidized CNFs exhibited cell viability exceeding the OECD-specified threshold of 50% in both models, confirming their classification as "nonirritant" under the Globally Harmonized System (GHS) criteria (Fujita et al. 2019). These findings strongly suggest that CNFs do not induce irritation to healthy human skin under the tested conditions.

5.4 Summary

Based on skin permeation and irritation studies conducted within the NEDO project (FY2017–2019), TEMPO-oxidized CNFs are unlikely to penetrate the skin and are classified as nonirritants. In permeation experiments, both chemically stained and fluorescently labeled CNFs applied to a 3D cultured human skin model were not detected within the skin layers or receptor fluid and remained confined to the outermost surface layer. This observation aligns with the well-established principle that substances with molecular weights exceeding ~500 Da are generally unlikely to penetrate the stratum corneum (Potts and Guy 1992; Sugibayashi 2007). CNFs are composed of multiple glucose units and have molecular weights far exceeding this threshold. These findings are consistent with previous studies and demonstrate the utility of CNF-specific visualization techniques developed in this study, which represent a novel methodological approach for future investigations of skin barrier function and nanomaterial safety assessment.

Nevertheless, further investigation is warranted to evaluate potential penetration under non-ideal conditions, including compromised skin barriers (e.g., wounds or abrasions) and appendageal routes such as hair follicles, sweat glands, and sebaceous glands. Skin irritation testing in accordance with OECD TG 439 confirmed the nonirritant nature of TEMPO-oxidized CNFs. Similarly, Kim et al. (2019) reported that CNFs were nonirritant in assays using 3D cultured human skin models. Furthermore, no cases of CNF-induced skin irritation have been documented in the literature to date.

Despite these reassuring findings, CNFs exhibit substantial variability in physicochemical properties depending on raw material sources, manufacturing processes, and surface functionalization. Accordingly, CNF-specific safety evaluations remain essential. In addition, CNFs are increasingly utilized in regenerative medicine and tissue engineering, particularly as wound dressing materials. However, their long-term biological effects remain largely unknown and warrant further investigation (Stoudmann et al. 2020). Our research has also confirmed the presence of bacterial and fungal contaminants, endotoxins, and β-glucans in CNF suspensions, underscoring the importance of comprehensive quality control in safety assessments (Horie et al. 2023; Fujita et al. 2023b, 2025a, b). Endotoxins, even at trace levels, exhibit strong biological activity and represent a critical consideration for products intended for internal use, such as those employed in regenerative medicine and medical devices (Tanamoto 2008).

Although current evidence indicates a low potential for adverse dermal effects, the safe use of NCMs in biological systems requires rigorous quality control and comprehensive safety evaluation encompassing detailed physicochemical characterization, biological response assessment, and long-term impact studies.

References

Fujita K, Obara S, Maru J, Endoh S, Kitano Y (2019) Evaluation of the effect of cellulose nanofibers on skin irritation using a 3D *in vitro* reconstructed human epidermis model. Toxicol Lett 314:S196–S197

Fujita K, Endoh S, Maru J, Sai T, Tomoko A, Goi Y, Obara S, Tani F, Yamamoto F, Ogawa T (2023a) A manual for toxicity testing of cellulose nanofibers. https://riss.aist.go.jp/results-and-dissemin/776/

Fujita K, Obara S, Maru J, Endoh S (2023b) Effects of advanced nanomaterials on the respiratory system of a murine COPD model. Toxicol Rep 11:481–492. https://doi.org/10.1016/j.toxrep.2023.11.009

Fujita K, Obara S, Maru J, Kawai Y, Endoh S (2025a) Pulmonary inflammatory responses and retention dynamics of cellulose nanofibrils. Toxicology 511:154038. https://doi.org/10.1016/j.tox.2024.154038

Fujita K, Obara S, Maru J, Endoh S, Kawai Y, Moriyama A, Horie M (2025b) Assessing cytotoxicity and biocompatibility of cellulose nanofibrils on alveolar macrophages. Cellulose 32(1):241–260. https://doi.org/10.1007/s10570-024-06238-4

Horie M, Fujita K, Endoh S, Sugino S, Maru J, Moriyama A, Ogura I (2023) Contaminant microorganisms in the *in vitro* evaluation of cellular responses of cellulose nanofibers and their microbial inactivation using gamma irradiation. Toxicol Mech Methods 33(9):741–754. https://doi.org/10.1080/15376516.2023.2238061

Hua K, Carlsson DO, Ålander E, Lindström T, Strømme M, Mihranyan A, Ferraz N (2014) Translational study between structure and biological response of nanocellulose from wood and green algae. RSC Adv 4(6):2892–2903. https://doi.org/10.1039/C3RA45553J

Kim SM, Ji Gwak E, Jeong SH, Lee SM, Sim WJ, Kim JS (2019) Toxicity evaluation of cellulose nanofibers (CNFs) for cosmetic industry application. J Toxicol Risk Assess 5:029. https://doi.org/10.23937/2572-4061.1510029

Lopes VR, Sanchez-Martinez C, Strømme M, Ferraz N (2017) *In vitro* biological responses to nanofibrillated cellulose by human dermal, lung and immune cells: surface chemistry aspect. Part Fibre Toxicol 14(1):1. https://doi.org/10.1186/s12989-016-0182-0

Nordli HR, Chinga-Carrasco G, Rokstad AM, Pukstad B (2016) Producing UltraPure wood cellulose nanofibrils and evaluating the cytotoxicity using human skin cells. Carbohydr Polym 150:65–73. https://doi.org/10.1016/j.carbpol.2016.04.094

OECD (2025) Test no. 439: *in vitro* skin irritation: reconstructed human epidermis test method, OECD guidelines for the testing of chemicals, section 4. OECD Publishing, Paris. https://doi.org/10.1787/9789264242845-en

Ong KJ, Shatkin JA, Nelson K, Ede JD, Retsina T (2017) Establishing the safety of novel bio-based cellulose nanomaterials for commercialization. NanoImpact 6:19–29. https://doi.org/10.1016/j.impact.2017.03.002

Potts RO, Guy RH (1992) Predicting skin permeability. Pharm Res 9(5):663–669. https://doi.org/10.1023/A:1015810312465

Stoudmann N, Schmutz M, Hirsch C, Nowack B, Som C (2020) Human hazard potential of nanocellulose: quantitative insights from the literature. Nanotoxicology 14(9):1241–1257. https://doi.org/10.1080/17435390.2020.1814440

Sugibayashi K (2007) Safety concerns of nanomaterials to skin: safety and skin penetration of nanomaterials. Fragr J 11:25–28. (in Japanese)

Tanamoto K (2008) Endotoxin and the quality control of medicine. Bull Natl Inst Health Sci 126:19–33. (in Japanese)

Chapter 6
Oral Toxicity: Experimental Findings and Safety Implications for Nanocellulose

Akihiro Moriyama

Abstract Cellulose nanofibrils (CNFs; also called cellulose nanofibers) and cellulose nanocrystals (CNCs) have potential applications in food products; however, unlike conventional microcrystalline cellulose, their oral safety remains unestablished. This chapter summarizes findings from published studies and the NEDO project regarding their oral effects. Overall, the available evidence demonstrates low acute and subchronic toxicity for both CNFs and CNCs, with 50% lethal dose values exceeding 2000–5000 mg/kg and no-observed-adverse-effect levels generally corresponding to the highest tested doses. Most studies report no treatment--related abnormalities in clinical signs, hematology, serum chemistry, organ weights, or histopathology. However, some investigations indicate physiological effects under specific conditions, such as altered nutrient absorption, changes in gut microbiota, or reduced body weight. Results from 28-day repeated-dose studies conducted under the NEDO project further support the low toxicity of mechanically fibrillated CNFs in rats and mice, with no pathological findings and only mild changes, such as slight body-weight reductions or decreased platelet counts. Beyond conventional toxicity endpoints, recent research highlights the importance of assessing gastrointestinal behavior and mucoadhesive properties. While current data suggest a level of safety comparable to that of conventional cellulose, additional long-term and nutritional studies are needed to support regulatory evaluation of nanocellulose for food applications.

Keywords Nanocellulose · Cellulose nanofibrils · Nanomaterial safety · Risk assessment · Safety assessment · Oral Toxicity · Nutrient Absorption · Gastrointestinal Behavior

A. Moriyama (✉)
Research Institute of Science for Safety and Sustainability (RISS), National Institute of Advanced Industrial Science and Technology (AIST), Tsukuba, Ibaraki, Japan
e-mail: moriyama-akihiro@aist.go.jp

I. Ogura, K. Fujita (eds.), *Nanocellulose Materials*,
https://doi.org/10.1007/978-981-92-2148-6_6

6.1 Introduction

Conventional microcrystalline cellulose is designated as generally recognized as safe (GRAS) by the U.S. Food and Drug Administration (FDA) for use as a food additive. However, cellulose nanofibrils (also referred to as cellulose nanofibers; CNFs), which are nanoscale materials, are not currently designated as GRAS, and reports on their oral toxicity remain limited.

The Organisation for Economic Co-operation and Development (OECD) has established several test guidelines (TGs) for evaluating the acute and subacute oral toxicity of chemical substances. For acute toxicity, these include TG 420 (Fixed Dose Procedure; OECD 2002a), TG 423 (Acute Toxic Class Method; OECD 2002b), and TG 425 (Up-and-Down Procedure; OECD 2002c). For subacute toxicity, TG 407 (Repeated Dose 28-Day Oral Toxicity Study in Rodents; OECD 2025a) and TG 408 (Repeated Dose 90-Day Oral Toxicity Study in Rodents; OECD 2025b) are specified.

This chapter presents an overview of the oral effects of CNFs and cellulose nanocrystals (CNCs), based on existing literature and findings from the NEDO project (FY2020–2024).

6.2 Information from Existing Literature

Table 6.1 summarizes published studies on the oral toxicity of CNFs and CNCs. Overall, these reports suggest that both CNFs and CNCs exhibit low oral toxicity. Key studies are summarized below and results obtained under the NEDO project (Yamashita et al. 2024a, b) are discussed in detail in Sect. 6.3.

Shimokawa et al. (2020) investigated the applicability of CNFs to food materials by preparing bamboo-derived CNFs via enzymatic pretreatment and bead milling of bamboo pulp. Acute oral toxicity was evaluated in mice according to OECD TG 420. CNF samples were prepared at dose levels ranging from 50 to 2000 mg/kg and administered via oral gavage to groups of five male and five female ICR mice. Following a 14-day observation period, necropsy was performed. No mortality was observed in any of the CNF-treated groups during the observation period, and no differences were found in general condition or body weight. Necropsy also revealed no abnormalities, and the LD_{50} (50% lethal dose) under the test conditions was confirmed to be >2000 mg/kg.

In a subsequent study, Shimokawa et al. (2021) conducted a 90-day repeated--dose oral toxicity study in rats to evaluate the long-term safety of bamboo CNFs. Bamboo CNF suspensions (1 wt%) were administered once daily via oral gavage to Crl:CD(SD) rats at doses of 50, 100, and 200 mg/kg/day, all administered at 20 mL/kg. Throughout the study, no deaths or CNF-related effects were detected in general condition, urinalysis, ophthalmologic examination, hematology, blood biochemistry, organ weights, necropsy, or histopathology. The no-observed-adverse-effect

Table 6.1 Oral toxicity studies of CNFs and CNCs

Test material	Animal	Administration period (OECD TG)	Dose (mg/kg/day)	Toxicity value	References
Bamboo CNFs	ICR mice	Single dose (OECD TG 420)	50–2000	LD_{50} >2000 mg/kg/day	Shimokawa et al. (2020)
Bamboo CNFs	Crl: CD(SD) rats	90 days	50, 100, 200	NOAEL ≥ 200 mg/kg/day	Shimokawa et al. (2021)
Lignin-coated CNFs and CNCs	SD rats	Single dose	5000	LD_{50} ≥ 5000 mg/kg/day	Ong et al. (2017)
Fibrillated cellulose from wood pulp	SD rats	90 days (OECD TG 408)	Male: 1044, 1550, 2194; Female: 1302, 1886, 2667	NOAEL ≥ Male: 2194.2 mg/kg/day, Female: 2666.6 mg/kg/day	Ong et al. (2020)
CNFs from softwood	Wistar Han rats	5 weeks, twice/week	100	CNFs have little acute toxicity and are likely nonhazardous when ingested in small quantities.	DeLoid et al. (2019)
CNFs from softwood	Wistar Han rats	5 weeks, twice/week	100	No associated pathology was seen within the duration of the study.	Khare et al. (2020)
CNFs from softwood	C57BL/6 mice	4–6 weeks	30	CNFs decreased the intestinal absorption nonspecifically, which might lead to nutritional risks after long-term exposure.	Chen et al. (2020)
Carboxymethylated CNFs	KM mice	8 weeks	1 or 3.5 w/w% (10 mL/kg)	No significant toxicity was observed.	Zhang et al. (2021)
CNFs from mechanically fibrillated pulp cellulose	Crl:CD(SD) rats	28 days (OECD TG 407)	50, 150, 500, 1000	Only female rats treated with 1000 mg/kg/day of CNFs exhibited a consistent reduction in body weight during the 14-day recovery period after the end of treatment.	Yamashita et al. (2024a)
CNFs from mechanically fibrillated pulp cellulose	C57BL/6JJmsSlc mice	28 days	400	No apparent toxic effects except for a slight decrease in platelet counts were observed.	Yamashita et al. (2024b)

(continued)

Table 6.1 (continued)

Test material	Animal	Administration period (OECD TG)	Dose (mg/kg/day)	Toxicity value	References
NCC™	Rats	Single dose (OECD TG 425)	2000	LD_{50} >2000 mg/kg	O'Connor et al. (2014)
NCC™	Rats	28 days (OECD TG 407)	500, 1000, 2000	NOEL >2000 mg/kg/day	O'Connor et al. (2014)
CNCs from wood pulp	SD CD® IGS rats	90 days (OECD TG 408)	Male: 1056, 1584, 2085; Female: 1278, 1930, 2683	NOAEL ≥ Male: 2085.3 mg/kg/day, Female: 2682.8 mg/kg/day	Ede et al. (2020)

level (NOAEL) under the test conditions was therefore determined to be ≥200 mg/kg/day.

Ong et al. (2017) evaluated the acute oral toxicity of lignin-coated CNFs and CNCs in female Sprague-Dawley (SD) rats. A single oral dose of 5000 mg/kg (volume between 0.91 and 0.98 mL) was administered as an initial limit test dose, followed by a 14-day observation period for mortality, gross signs of toxicity (including evaluation of skin/fur, eyes/mucous membranes, respiratory and circulatory systems, autonomic and central nervous systems, and somatomotor activity), and behavioral changes. Observations were made at 30 min and several hours postdosing, then once daily for 14 days. Body weight was measured on Days 7 and 14. At the end of the observation period, a gross necropsy was performed to examine tissues and organs in the thoracic and abdominal cavities. All rats survived and showed weight gain; no oral toxicity, clinical adverse effects, or behavioral abnormalities were observed. These results indicate that the acute oral LD_{50} for lignin-coated CNFs and CNCs exceeds 5000 mg/kg.

Ong et al. (2020) further assessed the 90-day dietary toxicity of fibrillated cellulose derived from wood pulp in accordance with OECD TG 408, comparing it with conventional cellulose (food-grade Solka-Floc). SD rats were fed diets containing 2%, 3%, or 4% fibrillated cellulose—corresponding to approximately 1044, 1550, and 2194 mg/kg/day for males and 1302, 1886, and 2667 mg/kg/day for females—for 90 consecutive days. The control group received Solka-Floc. Monitoring included survival, clinical observations, body weight, food consumption, ophthalmologic evaluations, hematology, serum chemistry, urinalysis, postmortem anatomic pathology, and histopathology. No adverse effects were observed at any dose level for either fibrillated or conventional cellulose in any of the measured endpoints. The highest tested doses—2194.2 mg/kg/day for males and 2666.6 mg/kg/day for females—were identified as the NOAELs for fibrillated cellulose. These results demonstrate that fibrillated cellulose behaves similarly to conventional cellulose and raises no safety concerns when used as a food ingredient at these concentrations.

DeLoid et al. (2019) investigated the effects of ingested softwood-derived CNFs under physiologically relevant conditions. CNF suspensions (average fiber diameter of ~50 nm) were prepared at 1 w/w% in either water or cream (20% fat) and administered via oral gavage to male Wistar Han rats at a dose of 10 mL/kg (~100 mg/kg CNFs) twice weekly for 5 weeks. Blood, serum, lungs, liver, kidneys, and small intestines were collected and analyzed. Although a reduction in body weight (30–40%) was noted in rats administered the aqueous CNF suspension compared with the other groups, the difference was not statistically significant. No significant differences were observed between groups in white blood cell counts (including neutrophils, lymphocytes, monocytes, eosinophils, and basophils), red blood cell counts, hemoglobin concentration, hematocrit, or other hematological parameters. Similarly, serum markers—including total cholesterol, HDL, total protein, albumin, liver function markers (e.g., total bilirubin), kidney function markers (e.g., creatinine), and electrolytes (sodium, potassium, chloride)—showed no significant differences between the CNF-treated and control groups. These findings suggest that ingested CNFs have little acute toxicity and are likely nonhazardous when ingested in small quantities.

In a related study, Khare et al. (2020) evaluated the effects of CNFs on fecal microbiome and metabolome, expression of epithelial cell adhesion genes, and cytokine production in the ileum under similar dosing conditions to DeLoid et al. (2019). CNF administration altered microbial diversity, reduced certain short-chain fatty acid-producing species, and increased insulin and IgA production. Furthermore, changes were observed in gene expression related to cell junctions and CD8+ T cell-associated immune responses. However, no pathological changes were detected.

Chen et al. (2020) administered softwood-derived CNFs (30 mg/kg/day; 3 mg/mL CNFs, 0.01 mL/g) or conventional cellulose to C57BL/6 mice in combination with a high-fat, high-sugar "Western diet" for 4–6 weeks. Control groups were administered either water + Western diet or water + standard diet. Both diets contained approximately 5% fiber, mainly in the form of conventional cellulose. Analyses included body weight, food intake, triglyceride levels, glucose homeostasis, intestinal absorption, and microscopic examination of the liver and gastrointestinal tract. Compared with the high-fat diet control group, CNFs decreased fat absorption in the jejunum and attenuated high-fat diet-induced fatty liver. However, a slight reduction in lean body mass and alterations in glucose homeostasis were observed. The CNF-treated group exhibited less severe fatty liver and fewer fat droplets compared with the group receiving conventional cellulose. Such results indicate that this dose of CNFs did not induce overt toxicity in mice but also suggest that CNFs may nonspecifically reduce nutrient absorption in the intestines, which could pose nutritional risks under long-term exposure.

Zhang et al. (2021) prepared carboxymethylated CNFs with varying carboxyl group contents (0, 0.36, 0.72, and 1.24 mmol/g) and characterized them based on morphology, diameter distribution, zeta potential, structural properties, rheological properties, suspension stability, and thermal properties. Aqueous CNF suspensions (1 or 3.5 w/w%) were administered orally to female KM mice once daily for 8 weeks at a dose of 10 mL/kg (approximately 100 or 350 mg/kg of CNFs). Body weight, food intake, and feces were monitored, and nutrient retention in feces was measured to assess the functional properties of CNFs. Blood and serum were also collected for analysis. Compared to controls, CNF-treated mice gained a significant increment in fecal fat, while food intake and body weight were significantly reduced by 10–15%. No significant differences were observed in hematology or serum markers between the control and CNF groups. These findings suggest that orally ingested CNFs are nontoxic and that carboxymethylated CNFs may be function as dietary components capable of reducing caloric intake by modulating lipid digestion and absorption in the gastrointestinal tract.

O'Connor et al. (2014) conducted a single-dose oral toxicity study and a 28-day repeated-dose oral toxicity study of CNCs in rats using NCC™, in accordance with OECD TG 425 and TG 407, respectively. No adverse effects were observed in general condition or pathological examinations in either study. The LD_{50} was determined to be >2000 mg/kg and the NOEL >2000 mg/kg/day.

Ede et al. (2020) conducted a 90-day repeated-dose dietary toxicity study in SD CD® IGS rats using sulfated CNCs derived from wood pulp, in accordance with OECD TG 408. CNCs were administered via the diet at concentrations of 0%, 2%, 3%, or 4%, corresponding to exposure levels of 1056, 1584, and 2085 mg/kg/day in males and 1278, 1930, and 2683 mg/kg/day in females, respectively. A control group fed conventional cellulose (food-grade Solka-Floc) at the same concentrations was also included. Standard parameters including clinical pathology, hematology, serum chemistry, urinalysis, necropsy, and histopathology were evaluated. No diet-related toxicity was observed in either the sulfated CNC or control groups. However, vacuolization around the hepatic portal area (with cytoplasmic vacuoles) was observed at the 4% dose in both groups, with comparable incidence and severity, and without associated liver function, degenerative changes, or pathological findings. Based on these results, sulfated CNCs were concluded to be safe for oral ingestion, similar to conventional cellulose, with a NOAEL of 2085.3 mg/kg/day for males and 2682.8 mg/kg/day for females.

Beyond conventional toxicity endpoints, several studies have evaluated the physicochemical properties, gastrointestinal behavior, and safety of fibrillated cellulose for potential food applications. For example, Pradhan et al. (2020) demonstrated through simulated digestion and toxicological evaluations that different types of fibrillated cellulose share consistent physical, chemical, and biological characteristics and that they do not induce adverse toxicological effects. Lin et al. (2019) showed that nanocellulose exhibits mucoadhesive properties in the gastrointestinal environment, with retention and adhesion depending on nanocellulose type, concentration, and gastrointestinal section, through mechanisms such as entanglement, gelling, or surface charge interactions. These findings highlight both the potential for broader applications of nanocellulose materials and the need to evaluate interactions with the mucus gel network.

Additional oral toxicity data for conventional cellulose (microcrystalline cellulose) are summarized in a report by the Joint FAO/WHO Expert Committee on Food Additives (JECFA 1998). No adverse effects were observed in three single-dose studies, with the LD_{50} values exceeding 3160 or 5000 mg/kg. Most repeated-dose studies found no histopathological abnormalities. JECFA concluded that toxicological data from both humans and animals do not indicate any potential toxic effects from consuming microcrystalline cellulose when used in food under good manufacturing practices.

Below is a summary of viewpoints from review articles:

In their review on recent developments and applications of CNCs in the food industry, Mu et al. (2019) highlighted that safety data is limited and there is currently no common regulation for nanocellulose. Stoudmann et al. (2020) reviewed the potential human health hazards of nanocellulose, including oral exposure to CNCs and CNFs, and concluded that, while the number of studies is limited and definitive conclusions are difficult to draw, no signs of toxicity have been observed to date. In a literature review evaluating the potential health risks of orally exposed nanocellulose, Brand et al. (2022) emphasized that animal testing data is limited and inconclusive. They highlighted key challenges, including variability in morphology and surface modifications, lack of standard reference materials, limited knowledge about intestinal fate and absorption, analytical difficulties in biological matrices, dispersion issues, and potential impurities or bioassay interferences. Vital et al. (2022) reviewed toxicological in vitro and in vivo studies of cellulose nanomaterials in food and biomedical applications and reported an increasing number of recent publications. Overall, ingested cellulose nanomaterials appear to be nontoxic to the gastrointestinal tract, with most tested materials demonstrating biocompatibility. However, they identified a lack of genotoxicity studies and long-term carcinogenicity or reproductive toxicity studies as a significant gap. Cañas-Gutiérrez et al. (2024) reviewed food applications and safety evaluations of nanocellulose and concluded that current toxicological studies do not indicate cytotoxicity or macrophage inflammatory responses. Nevertheless, the authors emphasize the need to establish intake limits and regulatory frameworks and highlight the importance of consensus on protocols and standardized test methods for safety evaluation.

6.3 Key Findings from the NEDO Project

Under the NEDO project, the University of Fukui conducted a 28-day repeated-dose oral toxicity study of CNFs derived from mechanically fibrillated pulp cellulose, in accordance with OECD TG 407 (Yamashita et al. 2024a). CNFs were administered via gavage to male and female Crl:CD(SD) rats at doses of 50, 150, 500, and 1000 mg/kg/day. Following the 28-day dosing period, the animals were observed for an additional 14 days to evaluate the potential reversibility of any toxic effects. Throughout the dosing period, no mortality was observed in either sex. Furthermore, no toxicological effects related to the test substance were detected in general clinical observations, functional observational battery assessments, urinalysis, hematology, blood biochemistry, necropsy findings, organ weight measurements, or histopathological examinations. Notably, female rats administered 1000 mg/kg/day exhibited a significantly lower body weight compared with the control group throughout the 14-day recovery period. In addition, pituitary gland and liver weights in these animals were significantly lower than those in the control group. However, no significant differences were observed in hematological or blood biochemical parameters, suggesting a potential weight-suppressive effect of CNF ingestion.

A separate 28-day oral toxicity study was also conducted in male C57BL/6JJmsSlc mice (10 animals per group) to assess the effects of repeated exposure (Yamashita et al. 2024b). The animals received mechanically fibrillated pulp-derived CNFs via gavage at doses of 0 or 400 mg/kg/day for 28 days (vehicle: sterile water for injection). The oral administration of CNFs for 28 days resulted in no apparent toxic effects except for a slight decrease in platelet counts.

6.4 Summary

This section summarized the findings from existing literature and the NEDO project regarding the oral effects of CNFs and CNCs. Across oral toxicity studies conducted in Japan and internationally, both CNFs and CNCs have consistently demonstrated low toxicity. For example, Shimokawa et al. (2020, 2021) reported no adverse effects in a 14-day oral toxicity study in mice and a 90-day oral toxicity study in rats using bamboo pulp-derived CNFs, even at the highest doses. In these studies, the LD_{50} exceeded 2000 mg/kg, and the NOAEL was at least 200 mg/kg/day. Similarly, Ong et al. (2020) reported that the NOAEL for a 90-day oral toxicity study in rats using fibrillated cellulose derived from wood pulp was at the highest dose tested, approximately 2000 mg/kg/day. Additional studies by DeLoid et al. (2019), Khare et al. (2020), Chen et al. (2020), and Zhang et al. (2021) likewise reported no significant toxicological effects following oral exposure to CNFs derived from softwood or carboxymethylated CNFs. In the 28-day oral toxicity study using rats conducted under the NEDO project with mechanically fibrillated CNFs, a significant reduction in body weight was observed in female rats administered 1000 mg/kg/day; however, no general toxic effects were identified (Yamashita et al. 2024a). Similarly, a 28-day oral toxicity study using mice revealed no abnormalities in body weight or gastrointestinal histopathology at a dose of 400 mg/kg/day (Yamashita et al. 2024b).

Although the number of available oral toxicity studies on CNFs and CNCs remains limited, the collective evidence from published literature and the NEDO project indicates no significant toxic effects. To date, no reports suggest that nanocellulose poses greater oral toxicity risks than conventional cellulose. Nevertheless, as noted by Chen et al. (2020), further investigation into nutritional aspects—such as effects on glucose homeostasis and intestinal nutrient absorption—is warranted to support safe food applications. In addition, important challenges remain, including addressing material diversity and impurities and conducting long-term studies on carcinogenicity and reproductive toxicity, which have not yet been undertaken.

References

Brand W, van Kesteren PCE, Swart E, Oomen AG (2022) Overview of potential adverse health effects of oral exposure to nanocellulose. Nanotoxicology 16(2):217–246. https://doi.org/10.1080/17435390.2022.2069057

Cañas-Gutiérrez A, Gómez Hoyos CG, Velásquez-Cock J, Gañán P, Triana O, Cogollo-Flórez J, Romero-Sáez M, Correa-Hincapié N, Zuluaga R (2024) Health and toxicological effects of nanocellulose when used as a food ingredient: a review. Carbohydr Polym 323:121382. https://doi.org/10.1016/j.carbpol.2023.121382

Chen Y, Lin YJ, Nagy T, Kong F, Guo TL (2020) Subchronic exposure to cellulose nanofibrils induces nutritional risk by non-specifically reducing the intestinal absorption. Carbohydr Polym 229:115536. https://doi.org/10.1016/j.carbpol.2019.115536

DeLoid GM, Cao X, Molina RM, Silva DI, Bhattacharya K, Ng KW, Loo SCJ, Brain JD, Demokritou P (2019) Toxicological effects of ingested nanocellulose in *in vitro* intestinal epithelium and *in vivo* rat models. Environ Sci Nano 6(7):2105–2115. https://doi.org/10.1039/C9EN00184K

Ede JD, Ong KJ, Mulenos MR, Pradhan S, Gibb M, Sayes CM, Shatkin JA (2020) Physical, chemical, and toxicological characterization of sulfated cellulose nanocrystals for food-related applications using *in vivo* and *in vitro* strategies. Toxicol Res (Camb) 9(6):808–822. https://doi.org/10.1093/toxres/tfaa082

Joint FAO/WHO Expert Committee on Food Additives (JECFA) (1998) Safety evaluation of certain food additives and contaminants. WHO Food Addit S 40. Microcrystalline cellulose. https://inchem.org/documents/jecfa/jecmono/v040je03.htm

Khare S, DeLoid GM, Molina RM, Gokulan K, Couvillion SP, Bloodsworth KJ, Eder EK, Wong AR, Hoyt DW, Bramer LM, Metz TO, Thrall BD, Brain JD, Demokritou P (2020) Effects of ingested nanocellulose on intestinal microbiota and homeostasis in Wistar Han rats. NanoImpact 18:100216. https://doi.org/10.1016/j.impact.2020.100216

Lin YJ, Shatkin JA, Kong F (2019) Evaluating mucoadhesion properties of three types of nanocellulose in the gastrointestinal tract *in vitro* and *ex vivo*. Carbohydr Polym 210:157–166. https://doi.org/10.1016/j.carbpol.2019.01.029

Mu R, Hong X, Ni Y, Li Y, Pang J, Wang Q, Xiao J, Zheng Y (2019) Recent trends and applications of cellulose nanocrystals in food industry. Trends Food Sci Technol 93:136–144. https://doi.org/10.1016/j.tifs.2019.09.013

O'Connor B, Berry R, Goguen R (2014) Chapter 10: risks, regulation, and management micro and nano technologies. In: Commercialization of cellulose nanocrystal (NCC™) production: a business case focusing on the importance of proactive EHS management, Nanotechnology environmental health and safety, 2nd edn. Elsevier, Cambridge, MA, pp 225–246

OECD (2002a) Test no. 420: acute oral toxicity—fixed dose procedure, OECD guidelines for the testing of chemicals, section 4. OECD Publishing, Paris. https://doi.org/10.1787/9789264070943-en

OECD (2002b) Test no. 423: acute oral toxicity—acute toxic class method, OECD guidelines for the testing of chemicals, section 4. OECD Publishing, Paris. https://doi.org/10.1787/9789264071001-en

OECD (2002c) Test no. 425: acute oral toxicity: up-and-down procedure, OECD guidelines for the testing of chemicals, section 4. OECD Publishing, Paris. https://doi.org/10.1787/9789264071049-en

OECD (2025a) Test no. 407: repeated dose 28-day oral toxicity study in rodents, OECD guidelines for the testing of chemicals, section 4. OECD Publishing, Paris. https://doi.org/10.1787/9789264070684-en

OECD (2025b) Test no. 408: repeated dose 90-day oral toxicity study in rodents, OECD guidelines for the testing of chemicals, section 4. OECD Publishing, Paris. https://doi.org/10.1787/9789264070707-en

Ong KJ, Shatkin JA, Nelson K, Ede JD, Retsina T (2017) Establishing the safety of novel bio-based cellulose nanomaterials for commercialization. NanoImpact 6:19–29. https://doi.org/10.1016/j.impact.2017.03.002

Ong KJ, Ede JD, Pomeroy-Carter CA, Sayes CM, Mulenos MR, Shatkin JA (2020) A 90-day dietary study with fibrillated cellulose in Sprague-Dawley rats. Toxicol Rep 7:174–182. https://doi.org/10.1016/j.toxrep.2020.01.003

Pradhan SH, Mulenos MR, Steele LR, Gibb M, Ede JD, Ong KJ, Shatkin JA, Sayes CM (2020) Physical, chemical, and toxicological characterization of fibrillated forms of cellulose using an *in vitro* gastrointestinal digestion and co-culture model. Toxicol Res (Camb) 9(3):290–301. https://doi.org/10.1093/toxres/tfaa026

Shimokawa T, Ikeda T, Magara K, Togawa E, Nakamura M, Otsuka Y, Nojiri M, Takao T, Ogawa M, Nakayama E, Hayashi N (2020) Cellulose nanofiber production from bamboo by enzymatic pretreatment for wet milling process using bead mill aiming at application to food materials. Bull For Forest Prod Res Inst 456:341–348. (in Japanese)

Shimokawa T, Magara K, Ikeda T, Hayashi N, Ogawa M, Takao T, Nakayama E (2021) Safety assessment of cellulose nanofibers obtained from soda cooking bamboo pulp: bacterial reverse mutation test, mouse lymphoma thymidine kinase assay, micronucleus test, and repeated dose 90-day oral administration in rats. Jpn Tappi J 75(11):1034–1050. https://doi.org/10.2524/jtappij.75.1034

Stoudmann N, Schmutz M, Hirsch C, Nowack B, Som C (2020) Human hazard potential of nanocellulose: quantitative insights from the literature. Nanotoxicology 14(9):1241–1257. https://doi.org/10.1080/17435390.2020.1814440

Vital N, Ventura C, Kranendonk M, Silva MJ, Louro H (2022) Toxicological assessment of cellulose nanomaterials: oral exposure. Nanomaterials (Basel) 12(19):3375. https://doi.org/10.3390/nano12193375

Yamashita Y, Tokunaga A, Aoki K, Ishizuka T, Fujita S, Tanoue S (2024a) A 28-day repeated oral administration study of mechanically fibrillated cellulose nanofibers according to OECD TG407. Nanomaterials (Basel) 14(13):1082. https://doi.org/10.3390/nano14131082

Yamashita Y, Tokunaga A, Aoki K, Ishizuka T, Uematsu H, Sakamoto H, Fujita S, Tanoue S (2024b) Assessing the safety of mechanically fibrillated cellulose nanofibers (fib-CNF) via toxicity tests on mice: single intratracheal administration and 28 days' oral intake. Toxics 12(2):121. https://doi.org/10.3390/toxics12020121

Zhang K, Zhang H, Wang W (2021) Toxicological studies and some functional properties of carboxymethylated cellulose nanofibrils as potential food ingredient. Int J Biol Macromol 190:887–893. https://doi.org/10.1016/j.ijbiomac.2021.09.055

Chapter 7
Emissions and Exposure: Case Studies and Strategies for Safe Handling of Nanocellulose

Isamu Ogura

Abstract Inhalation exposure, particularly in occupational settings, is widely recognized as a high-risk scenario for nanomaterials. This chapter focuses on airborne emissions and inhalation exposure associated with nanocellulose materials (NCMs), including cellulose nanofibrils (CNFs; also called cellulose nanofibers) and cellulose nanocrystals (CNCs). Existing literature on NCM emissions and exposure is briefly reviewed, followed by the presentation of case studies conducted under the NEDO projects, primarily targeting CNFs. These case studies include workplace measurements performed at CNF dry powder production and composite manufacturing sites, as well as simulated tests involving dry powder handling, droplet release from aqueous suspensions, and grinding or abrasion of CNF-containing composites. The findings indicate that dry NCM powders present the highest potential for airborne release and inhalation exposure, whereas aqueous suspensions are less prone to aerosolization and typically result in exposure to dried, aggregated particles. During grinding or abrasion of CNF-containing composites, most airborne particles consisted of resin fragments or resin–CNF mixtures, with CNFs remaining largely embedded and minimal direct exposure to isolated fibers. Based on these findings, key processes requiring attention, recommended countermeasures and management strategies, and practical measurement methods for emissions and exposure are summarized.

Keywords Nanocellulose · Cellulose nanofibrils · Nanomaterial safety · Emission assessment · Exposure assessment · Occupational exposure · Inhalation exposure · Workplace monitoring · Aerosol measurement · Dustiness test

---

I. Ogura (✉)
Research Institute of Science for Safety and Sustainability (RISS), National Institute of Advanced Industrial Science and Technology (AIST), Tsukuba, Ibaraki, Japan
e-mail: i-ogura@aist.go.jp

I. Ogura, K. Fujita (eds.), *Nanocellulose Materials*,
https://doi.org/10.1007/978-981-92-2148-6_7

7.1 Introduction

In general, the safety of chemical substances must be considered from both hazard and exposure perspectives. The occurrence and severity of adverse effects fundamentally depend on the magnitude and duration of exposure; therefore, appropriate exposure management is essential for the safe handling of chemical substances. This is particularly important when toxicological information is limited, in which case assessment and control of emissions and exposure become crucial.

Human exposure routes to chemical substances are broadly categorized into oral, dermal, and inhalation exposure. For nanomaterials, inhalation exposure—especially occupational exposure—is widely regarded as a high-risk scenario. Inhalation-related respiratory effects have been reported for various particles and fibrous materials, making inhalation exposure a major concern. For nanocellulose materials (NCMs), including cellulose nanofibrils (also referred to as cellulose nanofibers; CNFs) and cellulose nanocrystals (CNCs), which are characterized by fiber diameters in the nanoscale range (1–100 nm), inhalation exposure to dry powders is considered a high-risk scenario in the product lifecycle (Shatkin and Kim 2015). Accordingly, most existing studies on NCM emissions and exposure have focused on airborne emissions and inhalation exposure.

Accordingly, this chapter focuses on airborne emissions and inhalation exposure associated with NCMs. Prior to reviewing specific case studies, Sect. 7.2 provides an overview of occupational exposure limits (OELs) for various dusts to establish a general framework for interpreting workplace concentration levels. Although no OELs have been established specifically for NCMs, OELs for other nanomaterials and dusts provide useful reference values for voluntary exposure management. Section 7.3 summarizes existing research on NCM emissions and exposure, while Sect. 7.4 presents case studies of NCM emissions and exposure, with a primary focus on CNFs, conducted under the NEDO projects (FY2017–2019 and FY2020–2024). Finally, Sect. 7.5 provides a comprehensive summary of findings, highlighting critical processes, countermeasures and management strategies, as well as measurement methodologies.

7.2 Occupational Exposure Limits for Inhalation in the Workplace

7.2.1 Occupational Exposure Limits for Nanomaterials and Other Dusts

Figure 7.1 summarizes the recommended OELs for titanium dioxide nanoparticles (nano-TiO_2), zinc oxide nanoparticles (nano-ZnO), and various other dusts, as proposed by the Japan Society for Occupational Health (2024), as well as OELs for

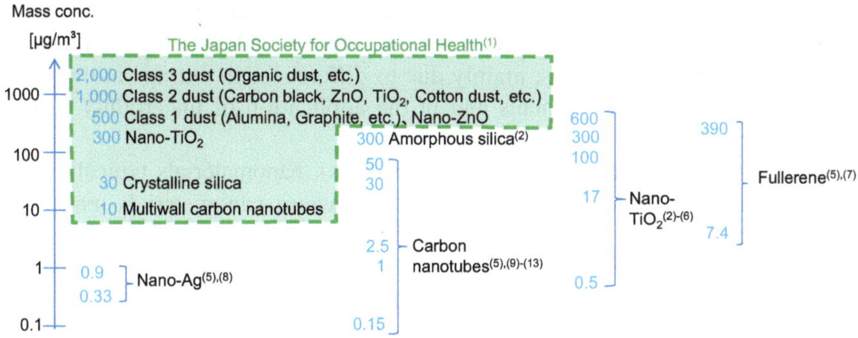

Fig. 7.1 Occupational exposure limits for nanomaterials and other dusts. (Sources: (1) Japan Society for Occupational Health (2024); (2) Stockmann-Juvala et al. (2014); (3) NIOSH (2011); (4) Gamo (2011); (5) Aschberger et al. (2011); (6) ANSES (2020); (7) Shinohara (2011); (8) NIOSH (2020); (9) Pauluhn (2010); (10) Nakanishi (2011); (11) NIOSH (2013); (12) Nanocyl; (13) Fukushima et al. (2018))

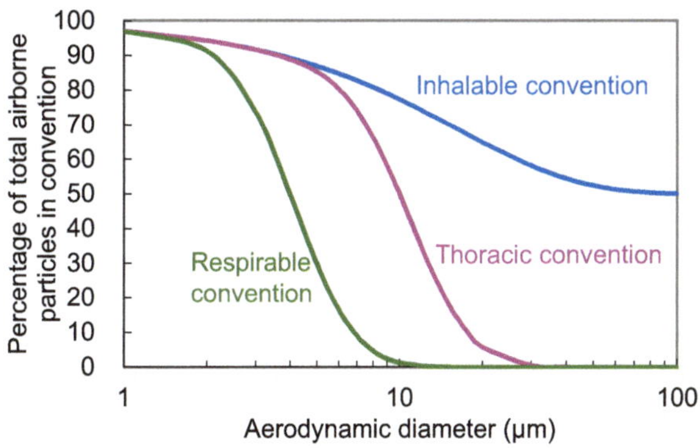

Fig. 7.2 Inhalable, thoracic, and respirable conventions expressed as percentages of total airborne particles as defined by ISO 7708 (ISO 1995)
Inhalable fraction: Mass fraction of total air-borne particles inhaled through the nose and mouth; Thoracic fraction: Mass fraction of inhaled particles, which penetrate beyond the larynx (50% penetration for 10 μm particles); Respirable fraction: Mass fraction of inhaled particles, which penetrate into the unciliated airways (50% penetration for 4 μm particles). The concentrations of inhalable, thoracic, and respirable dust refer to mass concentrations measured using samplers designed to achieve the particle collection efficiency shown above. For example, the respirable dust concentration is measured using samplers such as impactors or cyclones that remove coarse particles not entering the lungs, and are set to collect 50% of 4 μm particles

nanomaterials proposed by institutions and organizations in other countries. Although terminology and classification schemes differ among sources, these values are collectively referred to here as "OELs."

In occupational hygiene, respirable dust, defined by International Organization for Standardization (ISO) 7708 (ISO 1995) as particles with a 50% cut-off at a 4 μm aerodynamic diameter (Fig. 7.2), is commonly used as the basis for exposure assessment. Figure 7.1 primarily presents recommended OELs for respirable dust. Even for the same material, recommended OELs vary among institutions and organizations, mainly due to differences in extrapolation methods from animal data to humans and in the application of uncertainty factors (safety margins).

Compared with general dusts (Class 1–3 dusts), nanomaterials typically have relatively lower recommended OELs. This is because nanomaterials may elicit adverse effects at lower mass concentrations than larger particles. Several hypotheses suggest that toxicity may correlate more closely with surface area or bulk volume rather than with mass alone (Maynard and Kuempel 2005; Pauluhn 2011). However, because most toxicological studies for nanomaterials are conducted and evaluated based on mass concentration, the recommended OELs are also expressed in terms of mass concentration.

According to the Japan Society for Occupational Health (2024), non-nano titanium dioxide (TiO_2) and zinc oxide (ZnO) are classified as Class 2 dusts, with OELs of 1000 μg/m^3. In contrast, the OEL values for nano-TiO_2 and nano-ZnO are set at 300 μg/m^3 and 500 μg/m^3, respectively—approximately one-third to one-half of the values for their non-nano counterparts. Similarly, the U.S. National Institute for Occupational Safety and Health (NIOSH 2013) recommends an OEL of 2400 μg/m^3 for non-nano TiO_2, while the OEL for nano-TiO_2 is set at 300 μg/m^3, approximately one-eighth of the non-nano value. The British Standards Institution (BSI 2007) and the German Institute for Occupational Safety and Health (IFA 2009) propose applying benchmark values of $\leq$1/10 (for poorly soluble substances) to $\leq$1/5 (for soluble substances) of the OEL for the corresponding non-nano material when no nanomaterial-specific OEL is available.

Nanomaterials released into the air generally exist as aggregates or agglomerates. Most of the animal studies for deriving nanomaterial OELs were conducted using aggregated or agglomerated particles that are capable of reaching the lungs. Accordingly, these OELs can be considered as practically targeting aggregated/agglomerated particles.

Among existing OELs for dusts, asbestos represents a notable exception as its limit is defined based on fiber count rather than mass concentration. The British Standards Institution (BSI 2007) and the German Institute for Occupational Safety and Health (IFA 2009) have proposed the asbestos-based fiber count limit (0.01 fibers/cm^3) as a provisional benchmark for fibrous nanomaterials lacking established OELs. However, many fibrous nanomaterials, including carbon nanotubes and CNFs, are typically present as agglomerates and do not consistently exhibit discrete, countable fiber morphologies comparable to asbestos. In asbestos counting methods, agglomerated particles are excluded; only individual fibrous particles are included. Consequently, management of nanomaterials based on fiber count is often impractical. In fact, all currently proposed OELs for carbon nanotubes are based on mass concentration.

7.2.2 Occupational Exposure Limits for NCMs

At present, no OELs have been formally proposed for inhalation exposure to NCMs based on inhalation toxicity data. Based on the precautionary principle, the Finnish Institute of Occupational Health has proposed an OEL of 0.01 fibers/cm^3—the same value as that for asbestos—for NCMs and carbon nanofibers in the construction industry (Stockmann-Juvala et al. 2014). However, managing CNFs based on fiber count is generally impractical.

Although sufficient data on the chronic effects of inhalation exposure to NCMs are not yet available, short-term animal inhalation studies indicate that inflammatory responses induced by CNFs and CNCs are transient and comparable to those caused by conventional cellulose and other poorly soluble, low-toxicity dusts. These responses are markedly different from those induced by multiwalled carbon nanotubes (MWCNTs) or asbestos (Chap. 4). In intratracheal instillation studies conducted under the NEDO projects, inflammatory responses to CNFs diminished within 90 days and were substantially milder than those observed for MWCNTs (Chap. 4). Similarly, in intraperitoneal administration studies in mice, none of the three tested CNFs induced inflammation—a key initiating event in mesothelioma development—and no mesotheliomas were observed (Chap. 3). Taken together, these findings suggest that provisional workplace management concentrations for NCMs can reasonably be established by reference to OELs for conventional cellulose, other nanomaterials, and general dusts.

For non-nanoscale cellulose, the Japan Society for Occupational Health (2024) classifies cotton dust as a Class 2 dust, with OELs of 1 mg/m^3 for respirable dust and 4 mg/m^3 for total dust. For cellulose, NIOSH sets recommended exposure limits (RELs) of 5 mg/m^3 for respirable dust and 10 mg/m^3 for total dust, while the U.S. Occupational Safety and Health Administration (OSHA) sets permissible exposure limits (PELs) of 5 mg/m^3 for respirable dust and 15 mg/m^3 for total dust (NIOSH 2019).

As mentioned earlier, OELs for nanomaterials are generally set lower than those for their non-nano counterparts. Due to the lack of sufficient inhalation toxicity data specific to NCMs, it is therefore appropriate to manage NCMs at concentrations lower than those for conventional cellulose. BSI (2007) and IFA (2009) recommend applying a benchmark value of $\leq 1/10$ of the OEL for the corresponding non-nano substance for poorly soluble materials. Applying this approach to the respirable cotton dust OEL of 1 mg/m^3 yields a provisional benchmark of ≤ 100 μg/m^3. This value is slightly lower than the OEL values proposed for nano-TiO_2 (300 μg/m^3) and nano-ZnO (500 μg/m^3) by the Japan Society for Occupational Health (2024).

When establishing benchmark concentrations, practical measurability must also be considered. A dust concentration of 100 μg/m^3 is generally measurable via gravimetric analysis of particles collected on filters or by conventional dust monitoring systems. Furthermore, the national average concentrations of suspended particulate matter (SPM, ≤ 10 μm) and fine particulate matter (PM2.5, ≤ 2.5 μm) in Japan (general monitoring stations, FY2020; Ministry of the Environment 2022) are 14 and

9.5 μg/m^3, respectively. The attainment rate for the PM2.5 environmental standard (annual average ≤15 μg/m^3; daily average ≤35 μg/m^3) exceeds 98%, indicating that background particle concentrations rarely exceed 50 μg/m^3. Under these conditions, voluntary workplace safety management using a benchmark of 100 μg/m^3 for respirable dust is generally feasible, either by accounting for or subtracting background contributions.

If lower benchmark concentrations are adopted, it becomes necessary to distinguish and quantify (nano)cellulose separately from background particles. Although standardized measurement methods for cellulose in workplace environments have not yet been fully established, pyrolysis–gas chromatography–mass spectrometry (GC–MS) is considered a useful method for quantifying cellulose independently of background particles (Ogura et al. 2020a, b).

7.3 Information from Existing Literature

Although studies involving workplace measurements and simulated tests to assess NCM emissions and exposure remain limited, several evaluations using aerosol measurement instruments have been reported (Table 7.1). A summary of these studies is provided below. For reference, Table 7.2 outlines the main aerosol measurement instruments and their operating principles, while Fig. 7.3 illustrates the approximate particle size ranges targeted by each instrument.

Vartiainen et al. (2011) evaluated worker dust exposure during grinding and spray drying of microfibrillated cellulose (MFC). Measurements were conducted using a condensation particle counter (CPC) and a scanning mobility particle sizer (SMPS). Neither process resulted in significant particle exposure during normal operation. Grinding generated small amounts of particles; however, these were largely removed by a fume hood. During spray drying, particle leakage occurred when the duct valve was closed, but when the system was operated correctly, particle exposure was low or negligible.

NIOSH conducted measurements of dust emissions during various processes (Martinez et al. 2013; Geraci 2014; Glassford et al. 2020). Aerosol concentrations were monitored using CPCs, optical particle counters (OPCs), and dust monitors. For exposure characterization, cellulose labeled with cesium was employed, and cesium concentrations were quantified from filter-collected samples. During CNC slurry centrifugation, cesium was detected inside the cabinet (11.6 μg/m^3), just outside the cabinet (0.16 μg/m^3), and in the operator's personal breathing zone (0.14 μg/m^3), compared with a background concentration of 0.07 μg/m^3. During removal of the dried CNC product from a freeze dryer, cesium was also detected on the freeze dryer (0.016 μg/m^3), approximately two feet away from the product removed from the tray (0.03 μg/m^3), and in the operator's personal breathing zone (0.03 μg/m^3). In contrast, during removal of the dried CNF product from a freeze-dryer, cesium concentrations were below the quantification limit. During the production, cutting, and

Table 7.1 Studies on emission and exposure assessment of nanocellulose (existing literature)

Material	Measurement method	Target process	Results	References
MFC	Aerosol instruments (CPC, SMPS)	(1) Grinding (2) Spray drying	(1) Small amount of particles were generated, but they were mostly removed by fume hood (2) Particle leakage when duct valve was closed; minimal exposure during normal operation	Vartiainen et al. (2011)
CNFs and CNCs, both labeled with cesium	Aerosol instruments (CPC, OPC, dust monitor), filter collection of dust → Cesium analysis	(1) Centrifugation of CNC product slurry (2) Removal of dried CNC product from a freeze-dryer (general ventilation) (3) Removal of dried CNF product from a freeze-dryer (local exhaust) (4) Production, cutting, and milling of CNC polymer composite	(1) Cesium detected in all 3 samples: inside a cabinet (11.6 μg/m^3); just outside the cabinet (0.16 μg/m^3); in the operator's personal breathing zone (0.14 μg/m^3); compared with a background level of 0.07 μg/m^3 (2) Cesium detected in all 3 samples: on the freeze-dryer (0.016 μg/m^3), approximately two feet away from the product removed from the tray (0.03 μg/m^3), in the operator's personal breathing zone (0.03 μg/m^3) (3) Cesium below the quantification limits (4) Cesium detected in 6 out of 7 samples	Martinez et al. (2013), Geraci (2014) and Glassford et al. (2020)
Cellulose acetate nanofibers	Aerosol instruments (CPC, OPC, dust monitor)	Release of fibers from collection tank during production process	No detailed information	Glassford et al. (2020)
Nanocellulose	Aerosol instruments (CPC, OPC, dust monitor), filter collection of dust → SEM	Grinding, spray drying, particles escaping baghouse	No detailed information	Glassford et al. (2020)

(continued)

Table 7.1 (continued)

Material	Measurement method	Target process	Results	References
Nanocrystalline cellulose (NCC™)	Aerosol instruments (SMPS, OPC, TEOM)	(1) Spray drying/bagging (2) Cleaning of screw conveyor (3) Dustiness test using the rotating drum method	(1) OPC and TEOM concentrations increased to 2–3 times background; TEOM measured ~50 μg/m³ (2) OPC increased from 0.58 to 82 particles/cm³ when the system was opened for cleaning (3) The dustiness levels were moderate	O'Connor et al. (2014)
CNCs (5 spray-dried and 2 freeze-dried products)	Filter collection of dust → mass measurement	Dustiness test using the rotating drum method	The dustiness levels varied by CNC type and ranged from low to high	Ellis (2017)

Abbreviations: *CNC* cellulose nanocrystal, *CPC* condensation particle counter, *MFC* microfibrillated cellulose, *OPC* optical particle counter, *SEM* scanning electron microscope, *SMPS* scanning mobility particle sizer, *TEOM* tapered element oscillating microbalance (mass concentration measurement)

Table 7.2 Overview and principles of major aerosol measurement instruments

Instrument type	Overview/Principle
Optical Particle Counter (OPC)	Measures particle number concentration as a function of size (optical scattering diameter) for aerosols in the size range of ~0.3 to >10 μm (lower limit may be <0.1 μm depending on the instrument). Sample air containing aerosols is drawn through a laser beam, and scattered light from particles is detected. Because larger particles scatter light more intensely, particle size can be inferred from scattering intensity, while particle number is determined from the count of scattering events. However, the relationship between particle size and scattering intensity depends on the material's refractive index. As a result, particles with significantly different refractive indices from calibration particles (e.g., polystyrene latex) may yield inaccurate size readings. Many portable OPCs are commercially available for cleanroom use; however, in typical work environments they may exceed their upper concentration limit, leading to underestimation of particle count and overestimation of particle size due to multiple particles entering the detection zone simultaneously. OPCs designed for general environments with more size channels are referred to as aerosol spectrometers under ISO 21501-1. These use the same principle but typically measure only a portion of the sampled air to handle high concentrations

(continued)

Table 7.2 (continued)

Instrument type	Overview/Principle
Condensation Particle Counter (CPC)	Measures total particle number concentration for aerosols in the size range of approximately 0.01 to >1 μm (lower limit may be 0.001 μm depending on the instrument). Similar in principle to OPCs, but sample air is introduced into a supersaturated vapor (e.g., alcohol), causing vapor to condense on particles and enlarge them to detectable sizes. This enables detection of smaller particles that OPCs cannot measure. However, CPCs do not provide particle size information. Portable models are available and commonly used for general monitoring in workplace environments
Scanning Mobility Particle Sizer (SMPS)	Measures particle number concentration by size (electrical mobility diameter) for aerosols in the size range of approximately 0.01–1 μm (lower limit may be 0.001 μm depending on the instrument). Consists of a charger (e.g., neutralizer or corona discharge), a classifier (differential mobility analyzer, DMA), and a detector (CPC). Charged aerosols are introduced into an electric field in DMA, where particles exhibit mobility based on the balance between electrostatic force and fluid resistance, which depends on particle size. By adjusting the electric field, particles of specific sizes can be selectively measured. A single size distribution scan across the full particle size range typically requires several minutes. The electrical mobility diameter corresponds to the diameter of a spherical particle with equivalent diffusion properties
Aerodynamic Particle Sizer (APS)	Measures particle number concentration as a function of size (aerodynamic diameter) for aerosols in the size range of ~0.5–20 μm. APS operates on the principle that particle velocity after ejection from a nozzle depends on particle size. By measuring the time interval between two laser light scattering pulses as particles pass through dual laser beams, particle size is determined (smaller particles accelerate more and pass faster). Particle count is derived from the number of pulses
Dust Monitor	Measures approximate mass concentration of aerosols. Sample air is drawn through a laser beam and the total light scattering intensity from multiple particles is detected. Unlike OPCs, which detect individual particles, dust monitors measure the cumulative scattering intensity. Because mass concentration is approximately proportional to scattering intensity, the mass concentration is estimated from the scattering intensity. To improve accuracy, a mass concentration conversion factor—the slope relating scattering intensity to mass concentration—is determined in advance, for example, by performing simultaneous measurements with particle collection on filters

milling of CNC polymer composites, cesium was detected in six out of seven samples. In addition, NIOSH conducted workplace measurements using aerosol instruments at facilities manufacturing cellulose acetate nanofibers and other NCMs (Glassford et al. 2020).

O'Connor et al. (2014) evaluated potential dust exposure during spray drying and bagging of nanocrystalline cellulose (NCC™, the trade name for a specific CNC product) at the CelluForce demonstration plant. NCC™ is an aggregated powder with typical particle dimensions in the micrometer range. Aerosol measurements were conducted using an SMPS, an OPC, and a tapered element oscillating microbalance (TEOM, which measures mass concentration via a vibrating

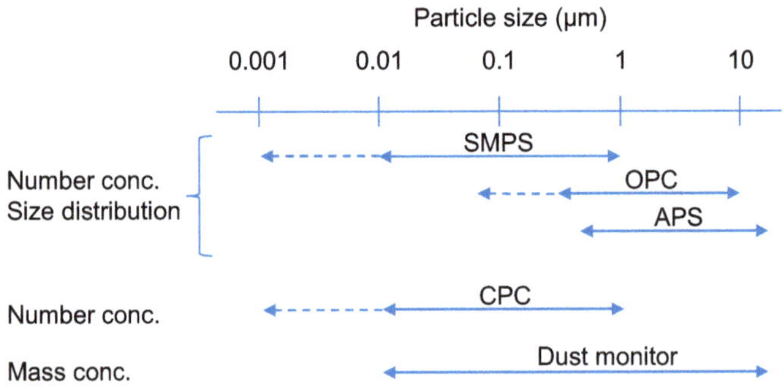

Fig. 7.3 Particle size ranges covered by aerosol measurements
Note: Particle size ranges are approximate and may vary depending on the specific product

microbalance element). During spray drying and bagging, concentrations measured by the OPC and TEOM—both sensitive to relatively large particles—were two to three times higher than background levels. It was noted that the plant was still in its initial start-up period and the bagging procedures had not yet been fully optimized. TEOM measurements indicated an overall particulate level of 50 μg/m^3, which are not considered particularly high in workplace environments. In contrast, SMPS measurements of nanoparticles showed little difference in nanoparticle concentrations between background and operational conditions.

Additional measurements were conducted during an upset condition in which the screw conveyor became clogged and the system was opened for cleaning. OPC readings increased from 0.58 to 82 particles/cm^3 when the system was opened but returned to near-background levels (0.74 particles/cm^3) once normal operation resumed. SMPS measurements showed higher nanoparticle concentrations under background conditions than during both upset and normal operation of the spray dryer, supporting the conclusion that the dried NCC™ aggregated powder is very stable and unlikely to release nanoscale particles during routine handling.

O'Connor et al. (2014) also assessed the dustiness of NCC™ using the rotating drum method in accordance with European standard EN 15051-2 (2013). Aerosol particles released during testing were classified into inhalable, thoracic, and respirable fractions (see Fig. 7.2 for definitions), and their mass was determined. NCC™ exhibited moderate dustiness across all three fractions, with inhalable dustiness values of 1241–1526 mg/kg, thoracic dustiness of 754–976 mg/kg, and respirable dustiness of 112–136 mg/kg.

Ellis (2017) evaluated the dustiness of five spray-dried and two freeze-dried CNCs using the same rotating drum method. Dustiness levels varied considerably depending on product type, with an inhalable dustiness range of 379–26,482 mg/kg, thoracic dustiness range of 134–8143 mg/kg, and respirable dustiness range of 10–970 mg/kg.

7.4 Key Findings from the NEDO Project

Workplace environment measurements and simulated tests conducted under the NEDO projects are summarized in Tables 7.3 and 7.4, respectively. Overviews of these studies are provided in Sects. 7.4.1 through 7.4.8.

7.4.1 Workplace Measurement at a CNF Dry Powder Production Facility

Workplace measurements were conducted at a CNF production facility, focusing on two operations: (i) collection of CNF dry powder following drying of the CNF slurry under ventilated airflow conditions, and (ii) transfer of the CNF dry powder from a large bulk bag into smaller bags inside a fume hood (Ogura et al. 2020b; Fig. 7.4). Airborne particles were monitored using CPCs, OPCs, and dust monitors. In addition, aerosol particles were collected on filters for gravimetric analysis, carbon analysis, pyrolysis-GC-MS, and scanning electron microscopy (SEM).

The results confirmed that CNF release occurred in both operations. However, the ventilation system and fume hood effectively prevented the released CNF powder from spreading into the workers' vicinity. The respirable CNF concentration near workers, quantified by pyrolysis-GC-MS, was below 2 $\mu g/m^3$. This level is sufficiently low when compared with occupational exposure limits for general dust and nanomaterials, such as carbon nanotubes and titanium dioxide nanoparticles (Fig. 7.1).

7.4.2 Workplace Measurement at a CNF Composite Manufacturing Facility

Workplace measurements were conducted at a ligno-CNF composite manufacturing facility to evaluate the potential release of CNFs and other particles (Ogura et al. 2020a). The evaluation focused on kneading (Fig. 7.5) and pelletizing (Fig. 7.6) of polyamide-6 (PA6)/ligno-CNF composites. For comparison, kneading and pelletizing were also performed using PA6 without CNFs (pulp). Kneading involves mixing resin and pulp using a twin-screw extruder under heat, during which the pulp cellulose is fibrillated to the nanoscale. The PA6/CNF composite underwent two kneading cycles. Pelletizing involves cutting extruded resin or composite strands into pellets of several millimeters. Airborne particles were monitored using CPCs, OPCs, and dust monitors, and collected on filters for gravimetric analysis, carbon analysis, pyrolysis-GC-MS, and SEM observation.

Aerosol measurements showed increases in particle concentration near the kneading equipment. Because these increases occurred both in the presence and

Table 7.3 Workplace environment measurements conducted under the NEDO projects

Material	Measurement method	Process	Results
CNF dry powder	Aerosol instruments (CPC, OPC, dust monitor), filter collection → gravimetric analysis, carbon analysis, pyrolysis-GC-MS, SEM	CNF dry powder production facility (1) Collection of dry powder (general ventilation) (2) Transfer of dry powder from a large bag into smaller bags (fume hood)	CNFs released during operations were effectively removed by the ventilation system or fume hood and did not spread near workers. The respirable CNF concentration near workers was below 2 $\mu g/m^3$, which is sufficiently low compared to general dust and nanomaterial exposure limits
Ligno-CNFs	Aerosol instruments (CPC, OPC, dust monitor), filter collection → gravimetric analysis, carbon analysis, pyrolysis-GC-MS, SEM	CNF composite manufacturing facility (1) Kneading (local exhaust ventilation) (2) Pelletizing	Aerosol concentrations during kneading and pelletizing were sufficiently low compared to existing dust and nanomaterial exposure limits
TEMPO-oxidized CNFs/liquid rubber powder	Aerosol instruments (CPC, OPC, dust monitor), filter collection → gravimetric analysis, carbon analysis, pyrolysis-GC-MS, SEM	CNF/rubber composite manufacturing facility (1) Recovery of dried CNF/liquid rubber powder (2) Kneading of CNFs/liquid rubber powder with styrene-butadiene rubber	(1) Near the sample outlet, the total dust concentration was approximately 100 $\mu g/m^3$. Repeated stirring under dry conditions, which is not normally performed, likely increased dispersibility. However, the respirable dust concentration was approximately 10 $\mu g/m^3$ or less (2) No clear concentration increase was observed

CNFs/triethylene glycol composite CNFs/polyester composite	Aerosol instruments (CPC, OPC, dust monitor), filter collection → gravimetric analysis, carbon analysis, pyrolysis-GC-MS, SEM	Cutting process of CNF composites	No clear difference in respirable dust concentration between idle operation and sample cutting, nor between near the cutting machine and the room entrance was observed. CNF respirable dust concentrations were estimated to be below a few μg/m^3. For total dust, concentrations were slightly higher during cutting than idle operation, and slightly higher near the cutting machine than at the room entrance. The maximum concentration was approximately 20 μg/m^3

Table 7.4 Simulated tests conducted under the NEDO projects

Material	Measurement method	Target process	Results	References
11 types of CNF dry powder and 1 type of CNC dry powder	Aerosol instruments (CPC, OPC, dust monitor, SMPS, APS), filter collection → gravimetric analysis, SEM	Simulated transfer of dry powder	The airborne particles released during the transfer process were approximately 0.1–10 μm in size. The amount of respirable dust released per sample mass was approximately 1–100 mg/kg. SEM observations revealed that the emitted particles did not appear as isolated fibers but rather as aggregated or agglomerated particles of several micrometers in size	Ogura et al. (2020a) and Ogura (in preparation)
8 types of CNF dry powder and 1 type of CNC dry powder	Aerosol instruments (CPC, OPC, dust monitor, SMPS, APS), filter collection → gravimetric analysis, SEM	Dustiness test using small rotating drum (EN17199-4 2019)	The released airborne particles were approximately 0.1–10 μm in size. The amount of respirable dust released per sample mass was approximately 10–300 mg/kg, and the number of released particles per sample mass was approximately 500–40,000 particles/mg	Ogura and Kotake (2026)

(continued)

Mechanical fibrillated CNFs, TEMPO-oxidized CNFs, phosphorylated CNFs	TEM, SEM	Evaluation of CNF aqueous suspension released as droplets	When droplets containing CNFs were captured before drying in the air, network-like CNF structures were observed. When dried in the air, densely aggregated particles formed due to droplet drying and shrinkage were observed	Ogura et al. (2020a)
Mechanical fibrillated CNF/PP composite, ligno-CNF/PP composite, ligno-CNF/PA6 composite	Aerosol instruments (CPC, OPC, SMPS), filter collection → gravimetric analysis, SEM	Grinding and abrasion tests of CNF composites	Airborne particles released during grinding and abrasion were similar regardless of CNF content. No fibrous particles presumed to be CNFs were observed. Most particles were considered to be resin fragments or resin-CNF mixtures. Similar results were obtained for aged samples	Ogura et al. (2020a)

Abbreviations: *APS* aerodynamic particle sizer, *CPC* condensation particle counter, *OPC* optical particle counter, *PA6* polyamide 6, *PP* polypropylene, *SEM* scanning electron microscope, *SMPS* scanning mobility particle sizer, *TEM* transmission electron microscope

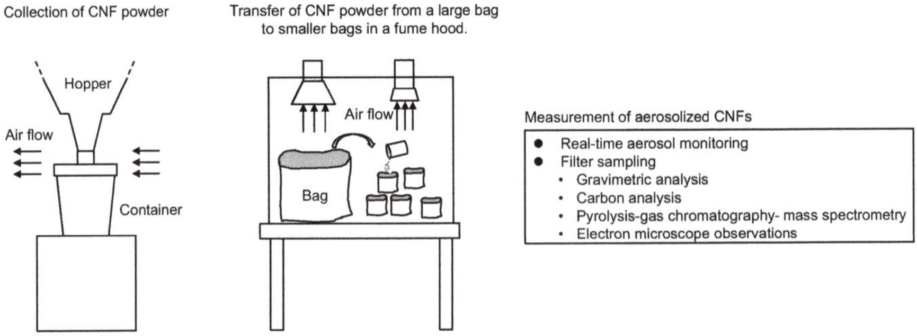

Fig. 7.4 Workplace measurements at a CNF dry powder production facility (Ogura et al. 2020b)

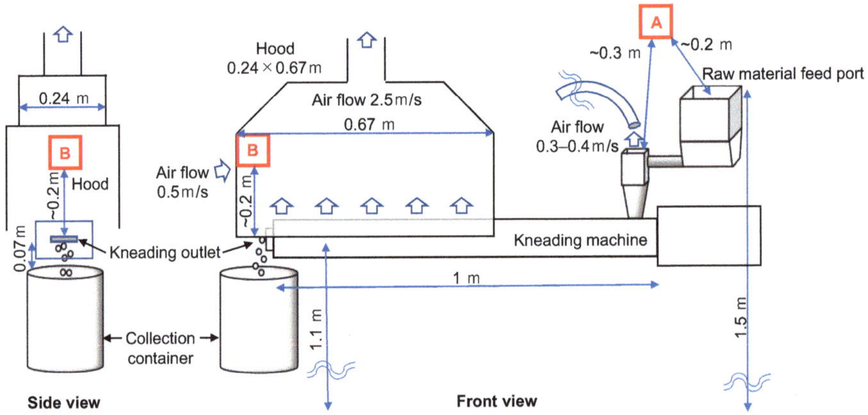

Fig. 7.5 Workplace measurements at a CNF composite manufacturing facility—kneading (Ogura et al. 2020a)
Measurement point A: near material inlet (approx. 20 cm from inlet); Measurement point B: near kneading outlet (approx. 20 cm from outlet) → Air primarily drawn into hood; Measurement point C: Control (approx. 4 m from kneading machine)

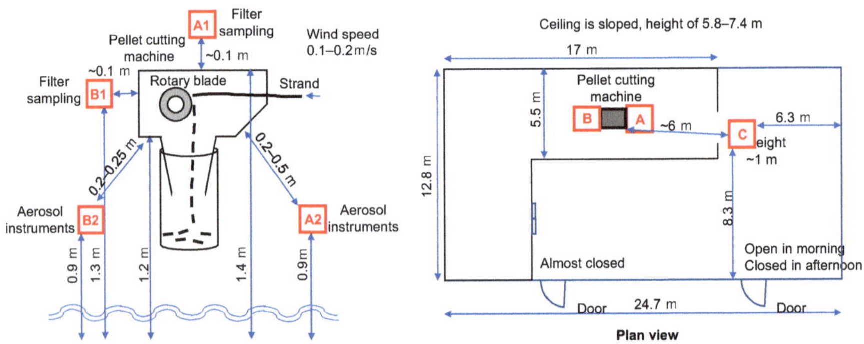

Fig. 7.6 Workplace measurements at a CNF composite manufacturing facility—pelletizing (Ogura et al. 2020a)
Measurement points A, B: near pellet cutter; Measurement point C: Control

absence of CNFs (pulp), they were attributed primarily to volatilized resin components generated during heating and machine operation rather than to CNF emissions. During raw material feeding, transient concentration increases were detected near the feed port, indicating limited dust generation; however, the total amount was small. No noticeable changes in particle concentration were observed before or after pelletizing.

Filter-collected aerosol particles were analyzed for total mass concentration by gravimetric analysis, carbon concentration by carbon analysis, and cellulose-equivalent concentration by pyrolysis-GC-MS. The total dust concentrations were slightly higher near the machines than at control points; however, no clear differences were observed between PA6 and PA6/CNFs operations. For respirable dust, cellulose-equivalent concentrations ranged from <0.7 to 9.5 μg/m^3 at control points and from 2.4 to 8.0 μg/m^3 near the machines, again showing no clear difference attributable to CNFs. These concentrations were well below occupational exposure limits for general dust and nanomaterials (Fig. 7.1). SEM analysis of filter-collected aerosol particles revealed no fibrous particles identifiable as CNFs or pulp fibers.

7.4.3 Workplace Measurements in a CNF/Rubber Composite Manufacturing Facility

Workplace measurements were conducted at a CNF/rubber composite manufacturing facility, focusing on two processes: (i) recovery of CNF/liquid rubber powder after drying (simulated using predried samples, followed by mixing and recovery operations; one cycle of approximately 5 min repeated 10 times; Fig. 7.7), and (ii) kneading of CNF/liquid rubber powder with styrene–butadiene rubber (from material feeding to recovery; one cycle of approximately 12 min repeated 6 times; Fig. 7.8). Airborne particles were monitored using CPCs, OPCs, and dust monitors, and were collected on filters for gravimetric analysis, carbon analysis, pyrolysis-GC-MS, and SEM observation.

During the powder recovery process, the total dust concentration near the powder outlet reached approximately 100 μg/m^3. Aerosol measurements indicated that repeated mixing under dried conditions—which does not represent typical industrial operation—led to progressively increasing airborne concentrations, suggesting enhanced aerosolization due to repeated handling. However, when limited to the respirable dust fraction, the concentration increase was restricted to approximately 10 μg/m^3 or less. In contrast, no appreciable increase in airborne particle concentration was observed during the kneading process.

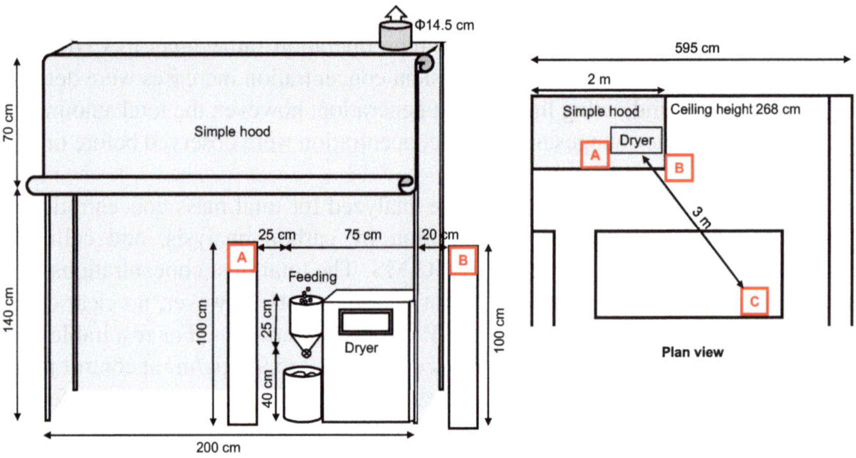

Fig. 7.7 Workplace measurements in a CNF/rubber composite manufacturing facility–recovery process of CNF/liquid rubber powder after drying
Measurement point A: near the powder outlet; Measurement point B: outside the simple hood; Measurement point C: Control (approx. 3 m from the outlet)

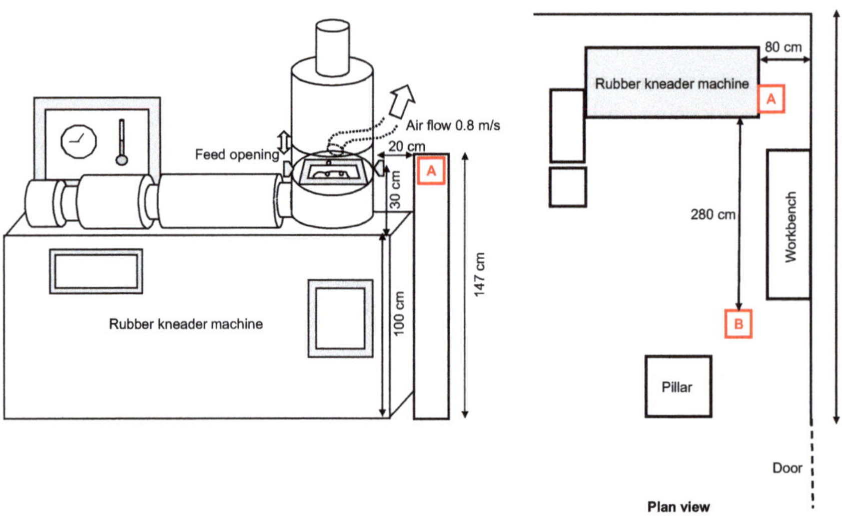

Fig. 7.8 Workplace measurements in a CNF/rubber composite manufacturing facility: Kneading process of CNF/liquid rubber powder with styrene-butadiene rubber
Measurement point A: near the sample feeding/removal port of the kneader; Measurement point B: Control (approx. 3 m from the port)

7.4.4 *Workplace Measurement During Cutting of CNF Composites*

Workplace measurements were conducted during cutting operations involving the following CNF composite materials (Fig. 7.9):

- CNF/triethylene glycol (TEG) dry composite (1:1.5),
- CNF/TEG dry composite (1:3),
- CNF/polyester composite.

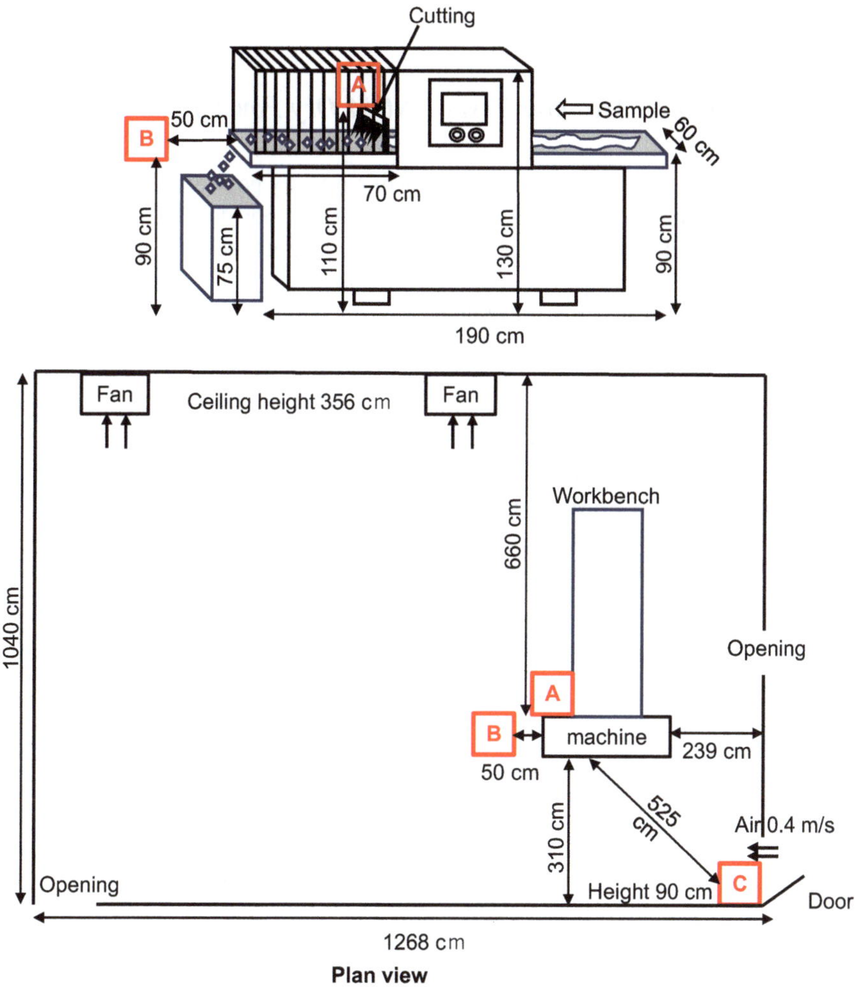

Fig. 7.9 Workplace measurements during cutting of CNF composites
Measurement point A: near cutting section of cutter; Measurement point B: near sample collection section; Measurement point C: Control (air inlet to room)

Airborne particles were monitored using CPCs, OPCs, and dust monitors, and collected on filters for gravimetric analysis, carbon analysis, pyrolysis-GC-MS, and SEM observation. Aerosol measurements revealed a slight but continuous release of submicron particles during cutter operation, along with brief emissions of micron-sized particles during postcutting cleaning. Filter sample analysis showed no clear differences in respirable dust concentration between idle operation and sample cutting, nor between near the cutting machine and the room entrance. The respirable CNF concentrations were estimated to be below a few μg/m^3. Total dust concentrations were slightly higher during cutting than idle operation, and slightly higher near the cutting machine than at the room entrance; however, the maximum concentration observed was approximately 20 μg/m^3.

7.4.5 Simulated Transfer Test of NCM Dry Powder

To assess aerosol generation during handling of NCM dry powders, simulated transfer tests were conducted using three types of CNF dry powder (Fig. 7.10) (Ogura et al. 2020a). Additional tests were performed using eight types of CNF dry powder and one type of CNC dry powder (Ogura in preparation).

The results confirmed that the released NCM particles were detectable using various aerosol instruments. The emitted NCM particles were approximately 0.1–10 μm in size. The amount of respirable dust generated per unit sample mass was approximately 1–100 mg/kg. Dust monitor readings were approximately 50–120% of airborne concentrations determined by filter collection analyses, indicating that uncorrected real-time measurements may either under- or overestimate actual concentrations. SEM observations revealed that the emitted NCM particles did not appear as isolated fibers but rather as aggregated or agglomerated particles of several micrometers in size.

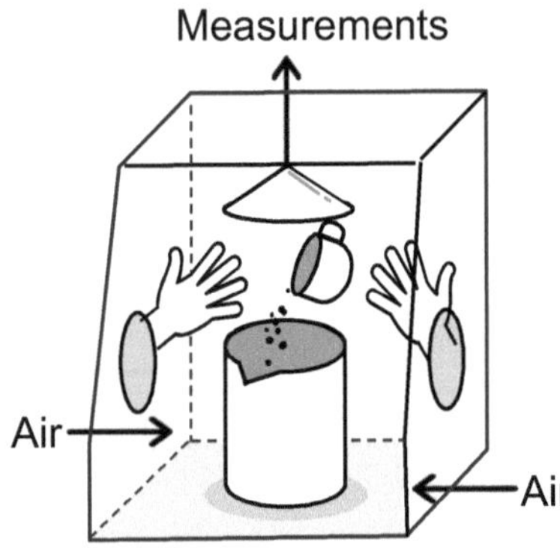

Fig. 7.10 Simulated transfer test of NCM dry powder

7.4.6 Dustiness Test of NCM Dry Powder

Dustiness tests were conducted using a small rotating drum (Fig. 7.11), following the European standard for evaluating the dustiness (aerosol generation potential) of powdered nanomaterials (EN17199-4 2019). The tests targeted eight types of CNF dry powder and one type of CNC dry powder (Ogura and Kotake 2026).

The emitted particles were approximately 0.1–10 μm in size, consistent with the simulated transfer test results. The amount of respirable dust released per unit sample mass ranged from approximately 10 to 300 mg/kg, while the number of released particles per sample mass ranged from approximately 500 to 40,000 particles/mg. These values were broadly comparable to those reported for titanium dioxide nanoparticles.

7.4.7 Dispersion of CNF Aqueous Suspension as Droplets

Release of CNF aqueous suspensions as droplets may occur during manufacturing (e.g., accidental ejection during production), product spraying, or leakage from the production lines. The aggregation state of CNFs in released droplets can vary depending on drying conditions, which may influence exposure levels and potential health effects. To investigate this behavior, CNF aqueous suspensions were emitted as droplets, and the morphology of deposited CNFs was examined under different drying conditions (Ogura et al. 2020a).

When CNF-containing droplets were collected prior to drying in air, network-like CNF structures were observed (Fig. 7.12, left). In contrast, when droplets were dried in the air, densely aggregated particles formed due to droplet drying and shrinkage (Fig. 7.12, right). In general, droplets larger than several tens of micrometers settle quickly due to gravity, whereas smaller droplets evaporate rapidly. Therefore, even if droplets containing CNFs are released into the air, inhalation exposure is expected to involve predominantly dried, densely aggregated CNF particles. Upon drying, CNFs strongly aggregate due to hydrogen bonding between

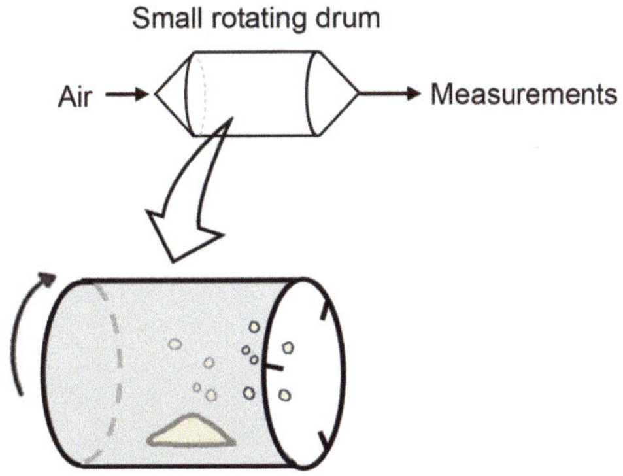

Fig. 7.11 Dustiness test of NCM dry powder

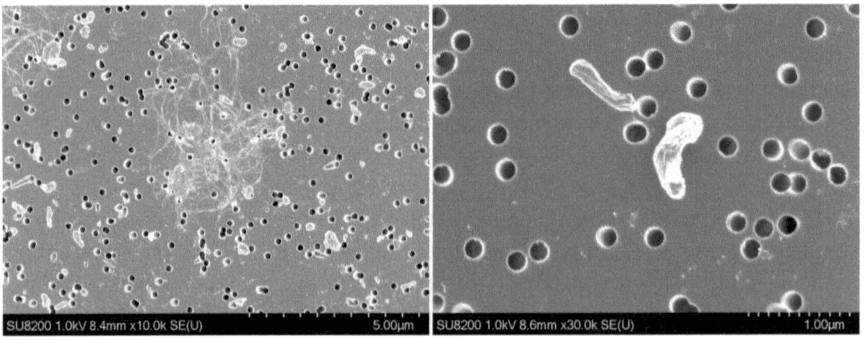

Fig. 7.12 CNF-containing droplets released into the air were captured before drying (left) and after drying (right) (Ogura et al. 2020a)

surface hydroxyl groups, leading to a reduced specific surface area. This behavior differs from that of other nanomaterials, such as carbon nanotubes or titanium dioxide, which may retain high surface area even in agglomerated states. However, under conditions of very high humidity where evaporation is suppressed, or when droplets consist of low-volatility liquids such as oils, exposure to fibrous CNFs in a dispersed state may still occur.

7.4.8 Cutting and Abrasion Tests of CNF Composites

To evaluate the potential for CNF emission and exposure during machining and abrasion of CNF composites, grinding and abrasion tests were conducted (Ogura et al. 2020a; Fig. 7.13). For comparison, resin materials without CNFs were also tested.

The particle size distribution of airborne particles generated during grinding and abrasion revealed no substantial differences between samples with and without CNFs. Morphological observations revealed no fibrous particles identifiable as CNFs. Instead, most airborne particles consisted of resin fragments or resin–CNF mixtures. Similar results were obtained in abrasion tests using aged samples. Although the available dataset is limited, these findings suggest that CNFs remain embedded within the resin matrix during machining and abrasion, and that direct emission or exposure to isolated CNFs is minimal. Dust generation occurs during grinding and abrasion irrespective of CNF content. However, by appropriately managing the emission and exposure of resin dust itself, emission and exposure of isolated CNFs can also be effectively controlled.

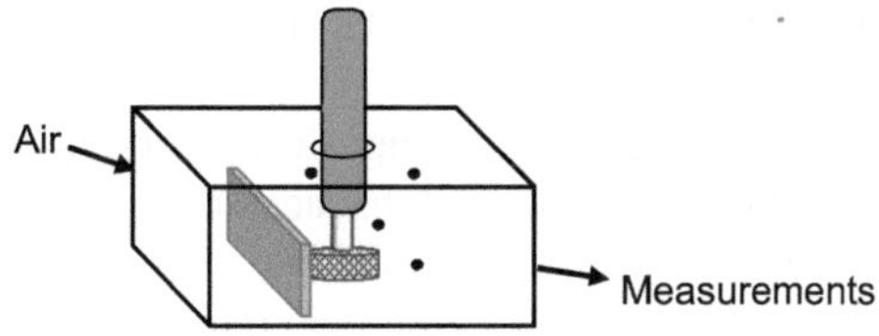

Fig. 7.13 Grinding and abrasion tests of CNF composites

7.5 Summary

This chapter focused on airborne emissions and inhalation exposure associated with NCMs, summarizing available information from existing literature. Although reports on NCM emissions and exposure remain limited, most studies are based on measurements using aerosol monitoring instruments. Under the NEDO projects, workplace measurements were conducted at CNF dry powder production facilities and CNF composite manufacturing sites, and airborne CNF concentrations were quantitatively evaluated using cellulose-specific analytical methods. In addition, various simulated tests were performed, including the handling of NCM dry powder, droplet release from CNF aqueous suspensions, and grinding/abrasion of CNF composites. Based on the findings, key processes requiring attention, recommended countermeasures and management strategies, and practical measurement methods for emissions and exposure assessment are summarized below.

Processes Requiring Attention from an Exposure Perspective
Handling of NCM dry powder tends to result in airborne particle release (O'Connor et al. 2014; Ellis 2017; Ogura et al. 2020a, b). Although NCMs are typically produced as aqueous suspensions, dry NCM powder is increasingly manufactured and distributed because of advantages in storage, transportation, and ease of handling during resin compounding. However, handling dry NCM powder poses a comparatively higher inhalation exposure risk and therefore requires caution. Similar precautions are necessary during cleaning and maintenance operations (Martinez et al. 2013; Geraci 2014; Glassford et al. 2020; O'Connor et al. 2014).

Compared with dry powder, NCM aqueous suspensions are less prone to becoming airborne and cause inhalation exposure. Nevertheless, potential release scenarios include ejection during manufacturing, spraying of NCM-containing products, or unintended leakage during manufacturing. Evaluations conducted under the NEDO projects demonstrated that when CNF-containing droplets were collected before drying in air, network-like CNF structures were observed, whereas densely aggregated particles formed when droplets dried in the air. These results suggest that CNF morphology at the point of exposure strongly depends on droplet drying behavior. In general, droplets larger than several tens of micrometers settle quickly due to gravity, while smaller droplets evaporate rapidly. Consequently, even when CNF-containing droplets are released into the air, inhalation exposure is expected to involve predominantly dried and densely aggregated particles. However, under conditions of very high humidity where droplet evaporation is suppressed, or when droplets consist of low-volatility liquids such as oils, exposure to fibrous CNFs may still occur.

Regarding CNF composites, workplace investigations conducted under the NEDO projects showed that aerosol concentrations during kneading and pelletizing were sufficiently low relative to existing OELs for dust and nanomaterials. Furthermore, airborne particle release during grinding and abrasion of CNF composites showed little difference between materials with and without CNF content. No fibrous particles identifiable as CNFs were observed; most airborne particles consisted of resin fragments or resin–CNF mixtures. Although the available data are limited, these findings suggest that CNFs remain embedded within the resin matrix, and that direct emission or exposure to isolated CNFs is minimal.

Recommended Countermeasures and Management Strategies
Ventilation and local exhaust systems, such as fume hoods, were shown to be effective in controlling released NCMs (Vartiainen et al. 2011; Ogura et al. 2020b). In particular, when handling dry NCM powder, the use of local exhaust systems and appropriate personal protective equipment is strongly recommended due to the high potential for airborne release.

Although no OELs have been formally established specifically for NCMs, provisional workplace management benchmarks can be derived by reference to OELs for other nanomaterials and dusts. OELs for nanomaterials are generally set lower than those for their non-nano counterparts. Accordingly, in the absence of sufficient data, managing NCMs at concentrations lower than those for conventional cellulose is prudent.

Following benchmark approaches proposed by the British Standards Institution and the German Institute for Occupational Safety and Health (setting OEL at $\leq$1/10 of the non-nano counterpart) an example benchmark for NCMs would be 100 μg/m^3, based on the 1 mg/m^3 OEL for respirable cotton dust. This value is slightly lower than the OELs for nano-TiO_2 and nano-ZnO (300 and 500 μg/m^3, respectively) proposed by the Japan Society for Occupational Health (2024). Furthermore, benchmark selection should also consider practical measurability in workplace environments.

During machining or abrasion of CNF composites, dust generation occurs regardless of CNF content. However, because CNFs are embedded within the resin matrix, direct release or exposure to isolated CNFs is expected to be limited. Consequently, effective management of resin dust emissions is likely to effectively control CNF exposure as well.

Practical Measurement Methods for Emissions and Exposure
Many studies have employed aerosol monitoring instruments such as CPCs, OPCs, and dust monitors. These instruments are compact and provide real-time measurements, making them suitable for routine workplace safety management. However, they cannot distinguish NCMs from other airborne particles. Therefore, comparative approaches—such as measurements with and without NCMs, before and during operations, near and far from emission sources, or relative to background concentrations—are essential.

For filter-based measurements, distinguishing NCMs from other particles remains challenging. For quantitative analysis of airborne cellulose, a method involving collection on quartz filters followed by analysis using pyrolysis-GC-MS is available (Ogura et al. 2020a, b). Although standardized measurement methods for NCMs in workplace environments have not yet been fully established, the case studies conducted under the NEDO projects (Sects. 7.4.1, 7.4.2, 7.4.3 and 7.4.4) may serve as useful references.

References

Aschberger K, Micheletti C, Sokull-Klüttgen B, Christensen FM (2011) Analysis of currently available data for characterizing the risk of engineered nanomaterials to the environment and human health—lessons learned from four case studies. Environ Int 37(6):1143–1156. https://doi.org/10.1016/j.envint.2011.02.005

British Standards Institution (BSI) (2007) Nanotechnologies—Part 2: guide to safe handling and disposal of manufactured nanomaterials, PD 6699–2

Ellis S (2017) Occupational health and safety characterization of several North American cellulose nanocrystals, Canada, 5–8 June. International Conference on Nanotechnology for Renewable Materials

EN 17199-4 (2019) Workplace exposure—measurement of dustiness of bulk materials that contain or release respirable NOAA or other respirable particles—Part 4: small rotating drum method

French Agency for Food, Environmental and Occupational Health & Safety (Anses) (2020) Expert appraisal on recommending occupational exposure limits for chemical agents, assessment of health effects for titanium dioxide under nanoform (nTiO2, P25). https://www.anses.fr/en/content/recommended-occupational-exposure-limits-titanium-dioxide-nanoparticles

Fukushima S, Kasai T, Umeda Y, Ohnishi M, Sasaki T, Matsumoto M (2018) Carcinogenicity of multi-walled carbon nanotubes: challenging issue on hazard assessment. J Occup Health 60(1):10–30. https://doi.org/10.1539/joh.17-0102-RA

Gamo M (ed) (2011) Risk assessment of manufactured nanomaterials: titanium dioxide (TiO_2). Final report issued on July 22, 2011. NEDO project "Research and Development of Nanoparticle Characterization Methods (P06041)". https://riss.aist.go.jp/en/research-outcomes/339/

Geraci CL (2014) Nanotechnology research at NIOSH delivering on the promise through responsible development. Cellulose nanomaterials: a path towards commercialization. https://www.nano.gov/sites/default/files/geracic.pdf

Glassford E, Neu-Baker NM, Dunn KL, Dunn KH (2020) Exposures during wet production and use processes of nanomaterials: a summary of 11 worksite evaluations. Ind Health 58(5):467–478. https://doi.org/10.2486/indhealth.2019-0169

Institut für Arbeitsschutz der Deutschen Gesetzlichen Unfallversicherung (IFA) (2009) Criteria for assessment of the effectiveness of protective measures. IFA. https://www.dguv.de/ifa/fachinfos/nanopartikel-am-arbeitsplatz/beurteilung-von-schutzmassnahmen/index-2.jsp

ISO (1995) ISO 7708:1995, air quality—particle size fraction definitions for health-related sampling

Japan Society for Occupational Health (2024) Recommendation of occupational exposure limits (2024–2025). Environ Occup Health Pract 6(1):ROEL2024. https://doi.org/10.1539/eohp.ROEL2024

Martinez KF, Eastlake A, Rudie A, Geraci C (2013) Chapter 1.2: occupational exposure characterization during the manufacture of cellulose nanomaterials. In: Production and applications of cellulose nanomaterials. TAPPI Press, pp 61–64

Maynard AD, Kuempel ED (2005) Airborne nanostructured particles and occupational health. J Nanopart Res 7(6):587–614. https://doi.org/10.1007/s11051-005-6770-9
Ministry of the Environment (2022) Air pollution status for fiscal year 2020. https://www.env.go.jp/press/110805.html (in Japanese)
Nakanishi J (ed) (2011) Risk assessment of manufactured nanomaterials: carbon nanotubes. Final report issued on August 17, 2011. NEDO project "Research and Development of Nanoparticle Characterization Methods (P06041)". https://riss.aist.go.jp/en/research-outcomes/339/
Nanocyl website, Working safely with Nanocyl products. https://www.nanocyl.com/expertise-center/health-safety-environment/working-safely-with-nc7000-and-nanocyl-formulated-products/
National Institute of Occupational Safety and Health (NIOSH) (2011) Current intelligence bulletin 63: occupational exposure to titanium dioxide. https://www.cdc.gov/niosh/docs/2011-160/default.html
National Institute of Occupational Safety and Health (NIOSH) (2013) Current intelligence bulletin 65: occupational exposure to carbon nanotubes and nanofibers. https://www.cdc.gov/niosh/docs/2013-145/default.html
National Institute of Occupational Safety and Health (NIOSH) (2019) NIOSH pocket guide to chemical hazards, cellulose. https://www.cdc.gov/niosh/npg/npgd0110.html
National Institute of Occupational Safety and Health (NIOSH) (2020) Current intelligence bulletin: health effects of occupational exposure to silver nanomaterials. https://www.cdc.gov/niosh/docket/archive/docket260a.html
O'Connor B, Berry R, Goguen R (2014) Commercialization of cellulose nanocrystal (NCC™) production: a business case focusing on the importance of proactive EHS management. In: Hull MS, Bowman DM (eds) Nanotechnology environmental health and safety, 2nd edn. William Andrew Publishing, Oxford, pp 225–246
Ogura I (In preparation)
Ogura I, Kotake M (2026) Dustiness and aerosol characteristics of nanocellulose powders: implications for workplace exposure and safety management. NanoImpact 41:100610. https://doi.org/10.1016/j.impact.2025.100610
Ogura I, Kajihara H, Kuboyama T, Oguri T, Kawamoto A, Gamo M (2020a) Examples of emission and exposure assessment of cellulose nanofibers and their applied products (in Japanese). https://riss.aist.go.jp/results-and-dissemin/776/
Ogura I, Kotake M, Kuboyama T, Kajihara H (2020b) Measurements of cellulose nanofiber emissions and potential exposures at a production facility. NanoImpact 20:100273. https://doi.org/10.1016/j.impact.2020.100273
Pauluhn J (2010) Multi-walled carbon nanotubes (Baytubes®): approach for derivation of occupational exposure limit. Regul Toxicol Pharmacol 57(1):78–89. https://doi.org/10.1016/j.yrtph.2009.12.012
Pauluhn J (2011) Poorly soluble particulates: searching for a unifying denominator of nanoparticles and fine particles for DNEL estimation. Toxicology 279(1–3):176–188. https://doi.org/10.1016/j.tox.2010.10.009
Shatkin JA, Kim B (2015) Cellulose nanomaterials: life cycle risk assessment, and environmental health and safety roadmap. Environ Sci Nano 2(5):477–499. https://doi.org/10.1039/C5EN00059A
Shinohara N (ed) (2011) Risk assessment of manufactured nanomaterials: Fullerene (C_{60}). Final report issued on July 22, 2011. NEDO project "Research and Development of Nanoparticle Characterization Methods (P06041)". https://riss.aist.go.jp/en/research-outcomes/339/
Stockmann-Juvala H, Taxell P, Santonen T (2014) Formulating occupational exposure limits values (OELs) (inhalation & dermal), scaffold public documents. http://scaffold.eu-vri.eu/filehandler.ashx?file=13717
Vartiainen J, Pöhler T, Sirola K, Pylkkänen L, Alenius H, Hokkinen J, Tapper U, Lahtinen P, Kapanen A, Putkisto K, Hiekkataipale P, Eronen P, Ruokolainen J, Laukkanen A (2011) Health and environmental safety aspects of friction grinding and spray drying of microfibrillated cellulose. Cellulose 18(3):775–786. https://doi.org/10.1007/s10570-011-9501-7

Chapter 8
Ecotoxicity: Methods, Challenges, and Findings in Assessing Ecological Effects of Nanocellulose

Rie Tai, Isamu Ogura, and Hiroyuki Mano

Abstract The increasing production and use of nanocellulose have raised concerns regarding their release into aquatic environments and associated ecological risks. This chapter reviews ecotoxicity research on cellulose nanofibrils (CNFs; also called cellulose nanofibers) and other nanocellulose, and summarizes key findings from the literature and the NEDO project. Previous studies indicate that CNFs exhibit low acute and chronic toxicity to aquatic organisms, including algae, crustaceans, and fish. However, growth inhibition has been reported in certain algal species at low concentrations under specific experimental conditions. Such variability is mainly attributed to differences in CNF physicochemical properties, production processes, dispersion stability, and test media composition, indicating the limited applicability of conventional guidelines to nanocellulose materials. To address these issues, CNF-specific analytical methods and ecotoxicity testing protocols were developed to ensure stable exposure conditions. Using these approaches, ecotoxicity tests were conducted on four representative CNF types. Most endpoints showed no adverse effects at concentrations up to 100 mg/L. Reduced reproduction of *Daphnia magna* was attributed primarily to decreased feeding efficiency rather than intrinsic CNF toxicity. Overall, ecological impact assessments indicate that the current ecological impact of CNFs in aquatic environments is low, while underscoring the need for additional chronic toxicity data.

Keywords Acute toxicity · Cellulose nanofibrils · Chronic toxicity · CNF quantification · Dispersion stability · Ecological risk · Growth inhibition · Immobilization · PNEC · Reproduction test

---

R. Tai · I. Ogura · H. Mano (✉)
Research Institute of Science for Safety and Sustainability (RISS), National Institute of Advanced Industrial Science and Technology (AIST), Tsukuba, Ibaraki, Japan
e-mail: r-tai@aist.go.jp; i-ogura@aist.go.jp; hiroyuki.mano@aist.go.jp

I. Ogura, K. Fujita (eds.), *Nanocellulose Materials*,
https://doi.org/10.1007/978-981-92-2148-6_8

8.1 Introduction

With the increasing practical application of nanocellulose materials (NCMs), their production volume and market distribution are expected to expand substantially. Consequently, the amount of NCMs entering aquatic environments via industrial and domestic wastewater is also likely to increase, raising the potential for exposure of aquatic organisms. It is therefore essential to assess not only the safety of NCMs for human health but also their environmental safety. Ecological risk assessments of NCMs provide critical information for guiding the development of applications with potential environmental release and for establishing appropriate disposal strategies.

In general, ecological risk assessments of chemicals and nanomaterials are based on ecotoxicity tests using representative aquatic organisms, including algae, crustaceans, and fish. These tests are typically conducted in accordance with internationally harmonized guidelines, such as those established by the Organisation for Economic Co-operation and Development (OECD). However, NCMs are poorly soluble in water and fall under the category of "difficult-to-test substances" as defined in OECD guidance documents. As a result, standard test methods based on OECD test guidelines (TGs) may not be suitable for accurately evaluating the ecological impact of NCMs (OECD 2019).

Under the NEDO project (FY2020–2024), existing literature on ecotoxicity tests of cellulose nanofibrils (also referred to as cellulose nanofibers; CNFs) was systematically reviewed, and current knowledge regarding their ecological effects on algae, crustaceans, and fish was compiled. In addition, key considerations from relevant OECD guidance documents were examined, and a comprehensive review paper was published to outline important points for establishing appropriate ecotoxicity testing methods for CNFs (Tai et al. 2022). Section 8.2 provides an overview of the current state of knowledge on NCM ecotoxicity tests, with a primary focus on CNFs, based on studies using algae, crustaceans, fish, and other aquatic organisms, drawing primarily on the aforementioned review. Section 8.3 introduces approaches for ecological risk assessment, including the derivation of predicted no-effect concentrations (PNECs) and their comparison with predicted environmental concentrations (PECs), based on multiple ecotoxicity test results, as reported by Stoudmann et al. (2019).

As summarized in the review paper, standardized testing methods for CNFs have not yet been fully established, and ecotoxicity studies are currently conducted using diverse, independently developed approaches. For example, CNFs tend to agglomerate and settle in the presence of medium components (e.g., salts), yet relatively few studies verify the actual concentration or dispersion state of CNFs in test solutions. Establishing ecotoxicity testing methods tailored to the physicochemical characteristics of CNFs therefore remains a key challenge. To address these issues, the NEDO project developed CNF-specific test methods and experimental conditions tailored to each CNF type under evaluation. Ecotoxicity tests were conducted according to these established protocols, and the resulting toxicity values were used to derive PNECs as indicators of potential ecological impact. The outcomes of these efforts are presented in Sect. 8.4.

8.2 Information from Existing Literature

This section summarizes ecotoxicity test results for NCMs, with a primary focus on CNFs, using algae, crustaceans, and fish, based mainly on the review by Tai et al. (2022). In addition, ecotoxicity tests on other aquatic organisms (e.g., shellfish) are also included.

To compile relevant information on laboratory-based ecotoxicity tests on NCMs using algae, crustaceans, and fish, a literature search was conducted covering publications from 2010 to 2021. The search employed the keywords "nano," "cellulose," and "toxicity," along with one of the terms "alga," "*Daphnia*," or "fish," using the PubMed database (https://pubmed.ncbi.nlm.nih.gov/). This search identified 10 papers for algae, 5 for *Daphnia*, and 10 for fish.

For publications from 2022 through the end of October 2024, the same search strategy was applied, and an additional 20 papers were identified via Google Scholar. Citation tracking of previously collected papers was also performed. After further screening, 13 studies reporting ecotoxicity tests on NCMs using algae, crustaceans, fish, and other aquatic organisms were selected for detailed analysis (Table 8.1). An overview of these studies is provided below.

Kovacs et al. (2010) conducted ecotoxicity tests on nine aquatic species using nanocrystalline cellulose (NCC) and carboxymethyl cellulose (CMC). The tests were performed in accordance with established guidelines or protocols as follows: rainbow trout according to Environment Canada (2000a); *Daphnia magna* according to Environment Canada (2000b); *Ceriodaphnia dubia* according to Environment Canada (2007); fathead minnow using the 3-week short-term reproduction test described by Kovacs et al. (2007); *Pseudokirchneriella subcapitata* using a 72-h growth inhibition test in 96-well microplates following Blaise and Vasseur (2005); a species of Anostraca according to International Organization for Standardization (ISO) 14380 (ISO 2011); and zebrafish using a 5-day embryo development test described by Hill et al. (2005). NCC affected fathead minnow reproduction at 290 mg/L and reduced rainbow trout cell viability by 20% at 34 mg/L, but showed little effect on other species at concentrations below 1000 mg/L. Overall, NCC was considered to have low potential toxicity and environmental risk.

Vartiainen et al. (2011) performed acute immobilisation tests with *D. magna* (OECD TG 202) using microfibrillated cellulose (MFC) and microcrystalline cellulose (MCC). At concentrations of 40–600 mg/L, neonate motility was inhibited by 15–25% for MFC and 15–35% for MCC, likely due to physical interference from particle adhesion rather than chemical toxicity.

Pereira et al. (2014) investigated the effects of cotton-derived CNFs on the growth of *Chlorella vulgaris* using Bold's Basal Medium with high ionic strength and water samples from the Seine River. CNF exposure significantly inhibited growth and cell viability at concentrations as low as 1 mg/L. Poor dispersion (absolute zeta potential values <30 mV) and extracellular polymeric substance formation around *C. vulgaris* cells were observed, suggesting physical blockage of nutrient uptake and gas exchange.

Table 8.1 Ecotoxicity data of nanocellulose materials

Test material	Test organism	Organism type	Endpoint	Toxicity value/Information	References
Nanocrystalline cellulose (NCC)	Rainbow Trout	Fish	Lethality	[LC_{50}] > 1000 mg/L (1,3,4), >10,000 mg/L (8)	Kovacs et al. (2010)
	Daphnia magna	Crustacean	Lethality	[LC_{50}] > 1000 mg/L (1, 2c), 250 mg/L (2a), 320 mg/L (2b), 210 mg/L (3), >5000 mg/L (4, 5a, 5b, 6, 7, 8, 9, 12)	
	Ceriodaphnia dubia	Crustacean	Lethality	[LC_{50}] > 1000 mg/L (1), 140 mg/L (2a), 320 mg/L (2b), 300 mg/L (2c), 160 mg/L (3), >5000 mg/L (4, 5a, 5b, 6, 8, 9, 12), 430 mg/L (7)	
			Reproduction	[IC_{25}] 200 mg/L (2c), >1000 mg/L (3, 4, 5a, 5b), 140 mg/L (6), >2000 mg/L (8, 10), 160 mg/L (9), >2000 mg/L (10)	
	Fathead Minnow	Fish	Reproduction	[IC_{25}] 290 mg/L (7)	
	Scenedesmus	Algae	Growth inhibition	[IC_{25}] 120 mg/L (4, pH: 2.3), >2500 mg/L (4, pH: 6.8)	
	Artemia species	Crustacean	Lethality	[LC_{50}] 3540 mg/L (4, pH: 2.3), >13,200 mg/L (4, pH: 6.8)	
	Zebrafish	Fish	Lethality, subacute/embryo development	[LC_{50}] > 6000 mg/L (8, 10), [IC_{50}] > 6000 mg/L (8, 10)	
	Rainbow Trout	Fish	Acute cytotoxicity	[EC_{20}] 34 mg/L (4), [EC_{50}] 245 mg/L (4)	
Microcrystalline cellulose (MCC)	*D. magna*	Crustacean	Swimming inhibition	15–35% inhibition at 40–600 mg/L	Vartiainen et al. (2011)
Microfibrillated cellulose (MFC)				15–25% inhibition at 40–600 mg/L	
Cotton-derived CNFs	*Chlorella vulgaris*	Algae	Growth inhibition	Significant growth reduction at all concentrations (1, 50, 100 mg/L) after 24 h in Bold's Basal medium; significant reduction at 50 and 100 mg/L after 96 h in Seine River water. Survival rate significantly decreased at all concentrations after 72 h in both media	Pereira et al. (2014)
Cotton-derived CNFs	Klebsormidium	Algae	Growth inhibition	Significant growth inhibition observed at all concentrations (1, 50, 100 mg/L) after 48 h; reduction in cell viability observed at various time points across all concentrations	Munk et al. (2015)

Chemically modified CNCs—8 types	Zebrafish (6-h postfertilization embryo)	Fish	Lethality, morphology	No significant effects observed at the highest tested concentration of 200 mg/L	Harper et al. (2016)
CNFs (Mechanical fibrillation, TEMPO Method)	Zebrafish (6-h postfertilization embryo)	Fish	Lethality, morphology	Among two types of CNFs from Forest Products Laboratory, mechanically fibrillated CNFs showed significant increase in mortality and yolk sac/pericardial edema at 250 mg/L; TEMPO-oxidized CNFs showed lower toxicity. CNFs from University of Maine showed no significant toxicity at 250 mg/L	
Lignin-coated CNFs	Scenedesmus	Algae	Growth inhibition	EC_{50} > 1200 mg/L, NOEC = 300 mg/L	Ong et al. (2017)
	D. magna	Crustacean	Swimming inhibition, mortality	EC_{50} > 6000 mg/L, NOAEL = 6000 mg/L	
	Zebrafish	Fish	Embryonic development, lethality, morphology	LC_{50} > 2000 mg/L	
Lignin-coated CNCs	Scenedesmus	Algae	Growth inhibition	EC_{50} > 2800 mg/L, NOEC = 175 mg/L	
	D. magna	Crustacean	Swimming inhibition, mortality	EC_{50} ~ 11,000 mg/L, NOAEL = 7000 mg/L	
	Zebrafish	Fish	Embryonic development, lethality, morphology	LC_{50} > 2000 mg/L	

(continued)

Table 8.1 (continued)

Test material	Test organism	Organism type	Endpoint	Toxicity value/Information	References
CNFs (from bleached undried softwood sulfite pulp via enzymatic pretreatment, mechanical shearing, and high-pressure homogenization)	*D. magna*	Crustacean	Mortality	No mortality observed at the highest tested concentration of 2060 mg/L (48 h)	Ogonowski et al. (2018)
			Reproduction (number of offspring, parental survival, time to first brood, body length of parent and offspring)	0.206 mg/L: Significant increase in parental body length 2.06 mg/L: Significant increase in cumulative and average number of offspring 20.6 mg/L: 3 of 12 parents died, no offspring, significant decrease in parental body length	
			Feeding rate	Slight stimulation of feeding observed at CNFs <1 mg/L and algae <0.9 mg C/L Feeding rate declined drastically at CNFs >1 mg/L or algae >0.9 mg C/L Maximum eightfold inhibition observed at 10–20 mg/L	
Carboxymethylated and fluorescently labeled CNFs			Gut evacuation time	CNFs content in gut decreased by >99% after 60 min; estimated half-life: 28 min	
Wood-derived CNCs, cotton-derived CNCs, and CNFs	*Scenedesmus* sp.	Algae	Growth inhibition	No effects observed at 10 mg/L for any endpoint. Oxidative stress observed at 0.01–0.1 mg/L in all three aquatic species tested	Wang et al. (2020)
	D. magna	Crustacean	Swimming inhibition		
	Zebrafish	Fish	Lethality		
CNFs (High-pressure homogenized)	Zebrafish (larvae)	Fish	Mortality, hatching, malformation, swimming ability	No effects on survival, hatching, or morphology observed across 0.1–30,000 mg/L. Exposure caused phenotypic effects such as inhibited neurite extension, axon guidance abnormalities, and motor neuron loss, resulting in reduced swimming ability.	Liu et al. (2020)
CNCs (Switchgrass-derived)				No effects on survival, hatching, or morphology observed across 0.1–30,000 mg/L. Fluorescent-labeled CNCs accumulated in embryo, brain, and trunk. Exposure caused phenotypic effects including inhibited neurite extension, axon guidance abnormalities, and motor neuron loss, resulting in reduced swimming ability.	

CNFs (Kenaf-derived)	*D. magna*	Crustacean	Swimming inhibition	$EC_{50} > 100$ mg/L	Pengiran et al. (2022)
	Zebrafish	Fish	Mortality	$LC_{50} > 100$ mg/L	
CNFs	*D. magna*	Crustacean	Swimming inhibition	Swimming inhibition was ≤14% at the highest concentration of 20 mg/L	Kokol et al. (2023)
CNCs				Swimming inhibition was 13% at the highest concentration of 20 mg/L	
Dialdehyde CNFs (CNF-ox)				Swimming inhibition was 14% at the highest concentration of 20 mg/L	
Dialdehyde CNCs (CNC-ox)				Swimming inhibition was 25% at the highest concentration of 20 mg/L	
CNF-ox-HMDA				56% swimming inhibition observed at the highest concentration of 20 mg/L	
CNC-ox-HMDA				$EC_{50} = 11.6$ mg/L; 85% swimming inhibition observed at the highest concentration of 20 mg/L	
Nonoxidized CNFs	Blue mussel	Bivalve	Uptake, sublethal biological responses (lysosomal membrane stability, neurotoxicity, oxidative stress, metabolism)	TEMPO-oxidized CNFs showed high bioavailability and were readily taken up by mussel tissues. Lysosomal membrane destabilization increased within 15–45 min at 0.001 mg/L exposure. Acetylcholinesterase activity significantly decreased at 0.001 mg/L. Gill activity decreased at 0.001 and 1 mg/L	Rusconi et al. (2024)
TEMPO-oxidized CNFs			Uptake, sublethal biological responses	Same as above	

(continued)

Table 8.1 (continued)

Test material	Test organism	Organism type	Endpoint	Toxicity value/Information	References
TEMPO-oxidized CNFs	European purple sea urchin (*P. lividus*)	Echinoderm	Egg fertilization, sperm motility, embryo development	No effects on intracellular ROS levels or fertilization competence at 1000 mg/L. Embryo development inhibition significantly increased at 1000 mg/L after 1-h exposure	Esposito et al. (2024)
TEMPO-oxidized CNFs	Another sea urchin species (*A. lixula*)	Echinoderm	Embryo development	No effects on intracellular ROS levels or fertilization competence at 1000 mg/L. Embryo development inhibition significantly increased at 100 mg/L after 1-h exposure	

Adapted from Tai et al. (2022), with modifications

Note: The symbol ">" indicates that no effects were observed at the highest tested concentration

In Kovacs et al. (2010), batch numbers are indicated in parentheses next to toxicity values

Abbreviations: *CNC* Cellulose nanocrystals, *CNF* Cellulose nanofibril or cellulose nanofiber, EC_{20} 20% Effective Concentration—concentration at which 20% of test organisms are affected, EC_{50} 50% Effective Concentration—concentration at which 50% of test organisms are affected, IC_{25} 25% Inhibitory Concentration—concentration at which 25% inhibition is observed, LC_{50} 50% Lethal Concentration—concentration at which 50% of test organisms die, *NOAEL* No Observed Adverse Effect Level—concentration at which no adverse effects are observed, *NOEC* No Observed Effect Concentration—concentration at which no effects are observed

Munk et al. (2015) studied the effects of cotton-derived CNFs on the filamentous green alga (*Klebsormidium flaccidum*). Growth inhibition and reduced cell viability were observed at all tested concentrations (1, 50, and 100 mg/L), with significant effects appearing after 48 h.

Harper et al. (2016) evaluated eight types of cellulose nanocrystals (CNCs) and three types of CNFs using zebrafish embryos to assess mortality, development, morphological abnormalities, and physiological functions. Most CNCs showed no significant effects at 200 mg/L. One type of mechanically processed CNFs showed increased mortality and edema at 250 mg/L, whereas other CNFs showed no toxicity. Observed differences in toxicity were potentially attributed to differences in mechanical processing methods, cellulose material source, end-product impurities related to purification methods and/or aspect ratio.

Ong et al. (2017) assessed lignin-coated CNFs (L-CNF) and CNCs (L-CNC) using algae, *D. magna*, and zebrafish embryos on three aquatic species. The no observed effect concentrations (NOECs) for algae were 300 mg/L for L-CNF and 175 mg/L for L-CNC, while the no observed adverse effect levels (NOAELs) for *D. magna* were 6000 and 7000 mg/L, respectively. The 50% lethal concentrations (LC_{50}s) for zebrafish embryos were both 2000 mg/L. No significant adverse effects were observed even at artificially high concentrations.

Ogonowski et al. (2018) examined the effects of CNFs on *D. magna* feeding, survival, growth, and reproduction. Acute toxicity tests showed no mortality at 2060 mg/L, although feeding inhibition was observed at concentrations above 1 mg/L. Moderate CNF exposure stimulated growth under low food conditions, whereas high concentrations adversely affected growth and reproduction due to food dilution effects. Fluorescently labeled CNFs were rapidly cleared from the gut, with a half-life of approximately 28 min and no evidence of translocation beyond the alimentary canal was observed. Wang et al. (2020) conducted growth inhibition tests on algae, acute immobilisation tests on *D. magna*, and acute toxicity tests on zebrafish embryos using CNCs and CNFs derived from wood and cotton. No acute toxicity was observed at 10 mg/L, although oxidative stress responses were detected at lower concentrations (0.01–0.1 mg/L).

Liu et al. (2020) investigated neurotoxicity of CNFs and CNCs in zebrafish embryos. While no dose-dependent mortality or malformations were observed, exposure resulted in motor neuron loss and impaired movement. CNFs and CNCs accumulated in embryos and altered gene expression related to neurodevelopment.

Pengiran et al. (2022) evaluated kenaf-derived CNFs and reported no swimming inhibition in *D. magna* neonates or abnormalities in zebrafish at 100 mg/L, in accordance with OECD TG 202 and TG 203.

Kokol et al. (2023) investigated the acute toxicity of dialdehyde CNF/CNC crosslinked with hexamethylenediamine (HMDA) in *D. magna* neonates. At 20 mg/L, CNC-ox-HMDA caused 85% swimming inhibition, while CNF-ox-HMDA caused 56%. Toxicity was linked to surface chemistry and particle size, affecting adhesion to *D. magna*.

Rusconi et al. (2024) evaluated the acute toxicity of TEMPO-oxidized and non-oxidized CNFs in marine mussels. CNFs were detected in gill and hemolymph tissues, causing lysosomal membrane destabilization and inhibition of P-glycoprotein activity. Even under environmentally realistic exposure scenarios, CNF uptake and immune disruption were observed.

Esposito et al. (2024) assessed the environmental safety of leachates from nanostructured cellulose sponges (CNS) on the reproduction of two sea-urchin species (*Arbacia lixula* and *Paracentrotus lividus*). TEMPO-oxidized CNFs, as a constituent of CNS, reduced normal larval development at 100 mg/L in *A. lixula* and 1000 mg/L in *P. lividus*, but did not affect fertilization competence.

The relationship between CNF concentration and its effects on key endpoints for each biological species is summarized in Table 8.2. For algae, two studies reported effects at the lowest tested concentration of 1 mg/L (Pereira et al. 2014; Munk et al. 2015), suggesting that algae may be more sensitive to CNF exposure than other taxa. In contrast, other studies on algae reported no observable effects even at higher concentrations (Wang et al. 2020; Ong et al. 2017).

In acute toxicity tests on *D. magna*, slight swimming inhibition was reported at concentrations of 20–40 mg/L (Kokol et al. 2023; Vartiainen et al. 2011), whereas multiple studies reported no effects even at the highest tested concentrations (Wang et al. 2020; Pengiran et al. 2022; Ogonowski et al. 2018; Ong et al. 2017). Only one study provided chronic toxicity data for *D. magna*, reporting a lowest observed adverse effect level (LOAEL) of 20.6 mg/L and a NOAEL of 2.06 mg/L (Ogonowski et al. 2018).

For zebrafish, one study reported a significant increase in mortality and the occurrence of yolk sac and pericardial edema at 250 mg/L (Harper et al. 2016). However, in the same study, two other types of CNFs showed no observable effects even at 250 mg/L. Numerous additional studies likewise reported no effects at the highest tested concentrations (Wang et al. 2020; Pengiran et al. 2022; Harper et al. 2016; Ong et al. 2017; Liu et al. 2020).

According to OECD TGs, when a test chemical is expected to exhibit low or no toxicity, limit tests can be performed for *D. magna* reproduction at a test concentration of 10 mg/L (OECD 2012) and at 100 mg/L for *D. magna* immobilization and fish survival (OECD 2004, 2025a). Many CNF-related studies on *D. magna* and fish were conducted at concentrations exceeding these OECD limit test thresholds, and still reported no observable effects. Taken together, these findings suggest that CNFs generally exhibit low toxicity to aquatic organisms compared with typical chemical substances.

8.3 Ecological Risk Assessment of NCMs

At present, the production volume of NCMs, both domestically and internationally, is not at a level that raises concerns regarding environmental release or ecological impact. However, considering the potential for future expansion of NCM production, it is desirable for manufacturers to be able to predict and assess potential

Table 8.2 Summary of observed effect concentrations for key endpoints in aquatic species

Species (Endpoint)	References	Test material	Effect observed	CNF concentration [mg/L]	OECD TG No.
Algae (Chronic Toxicity: Growth Inhibition)[a]	Pereira et al. (2014)	Cotton-derived CNFs	**Yes**	**<1**	
	Munk et al. (2015)	Cotton-derived CNFs	**Yes**	**<1**	
	Wang et al. (2020)	Cotton-derived CNFs	No	>10	201
	Ong et al. (2017)	Lignin-coated CNFs	No	300	201
Daphnia magna (Acute Toxicity: Swimming Inhibition, Mortality)	Kokol et al. (2023)	Mechanically fibrillated CNFs	**Yes (≤14%)**	**20**	
	Vartiainen et al. (2011)	MFC	**Yes (15–25%)**	**40–600**	202
	Wang et al. (2020)	Cotton-derived CNFs	No	>10	202
	Pengiran et al. (2022)	Kenaf-derived CNFs	No	>100	
	Ogonowski et al. (2018)	Mechanically fibrillated CNFs	No	>2060	202
	Ong et al. (2017)	Lignin-coated CNFs	No	>6000	202
Daphnia magna (Chronic Toxicity: Reproduction)	Ogonowski et al. (2018)	Mechanically fibrillated CNFs	No	2.06	211
			Yes	**20.6**	
Zebrafish (Acute Toxicity: Mortality, Embryo Development, Morphology)	Harper et al. (2016)	Mechanically fibrillated CNFs	**Yes**	**250**	
	Wang et al. (2020)	Cotton-derived CNFs	No	>10	236
	Pengiran et al. (2022)	Kenaf-derived CNFs	No	>100	
	Harper et al. (2016)	Mechanically fibrillated CNFs	No	>250	
	Harper et al. (2016)	TEMPO--oxidized CNFs	No	>250	
	Ong et al. (2017)	Lignin-coated CNFs	No	>2000	
	Liu et al. (2020)	Mechanically fibrillated CNFs	No	>30,000	

“>” indicates that no effects were observed even at the highest tested concentration
“<” indicates that effects were observed even at the lowest tested concentration
[a]The results shown for algae are based on a chronic toxicity assessment method that compares growth rates between control and treatment groups to derive the no observed effect concentration (NOEC) value

ecological risks associated with NCM release into the environment from industrial sites in order to ensure safety.

In general, ecological risk assessment involves two key processes:

- Exposure assessment, which estimates the concentration of a substance in the environment, and.
- Ecological effect (hazard) assessment, which quantifies the harmful effects on organisms or biological communities.

These assessments aim to derive the following parameters:

- Predicted environmental concentration (PEC) from the exposure assessment, and
- Predicted no-effect concentration (PNEC) from the hazard assessment.

For typical chemical substances, PEC is estimated based on production volumes and measured environmental concentrations. Regarding NCMs, however, data on environmental release and environmental concentrations are currently unavailable. Moreover, because cellulose is a natural component of plants and widely present in the environment, it is extremely difficult to distinguish anthropogenically released NCMs from naturally occurring cellulose once released. Similarly, as discussed in Sect. 8.2, the ecotoxicity database required for robust PNEC derivation remains limited.

To address these challenges, Stoudmann et al. (2019) performed an ecological risk assessment using the following probabilistic approaches:

- Dynamic probabilistic material flow analysis (DPMFA) to estimate PEC, and
- Probabilistic species sensitivity distribution (PSSD) to derive PNEC.

Species sensitivity distribution (SSD) analysis is a commonly used method in ecological risk assessment, based on the empirical assumption that species sensitivities to a substance follow a statistical distribution. SSD describes the variability in sensitivity across different species as a distribution curve.

A key feature of these probabilistic methods is that both PEC and PNEC are expressed as probability distributions rather than single point estimates. Figure 8.1 illustrates the conceptual framework of this probabilistic risk assessment approach.

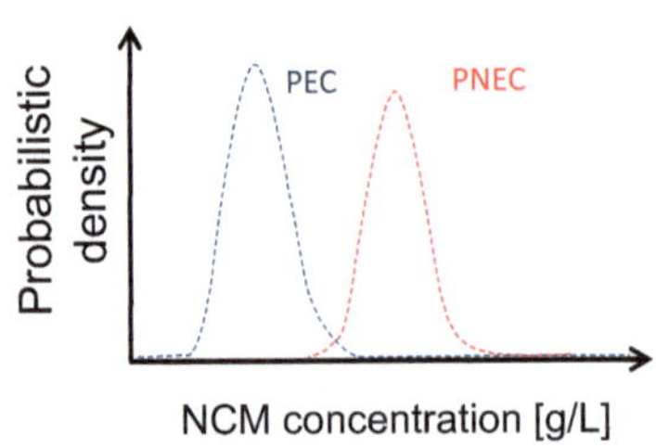

Fig. 8.1 Conceptual diagram of probabilistic risk assessment
The overlapping area between the PEC distribution, calculated via dynamic probabilistic material flow analysis, and the PNEC distribution, derived from probabilistic species sensitivity distribution, represents the risk characterization ratio (RCR)

The area of overlap between the PEC and PNEC distributions represents the risk characterization ratio (RCR). When no overlap exists between the distributions, the ecological risk is considered negligible or nonexistent.

This section provides an overview of the methods and results used by Stoudmann et al. (2019) to derive PEC and PNEC.

8.3.1 Calculation of PEC

Stoudmann et al. (2019) assessed NCM production and environmental release in Europe from 2000 to 2025. First, parameters required for DPMFA were collected from existing literature, including market research reports forecasting future production volumes. These data were then allocated to environmental compartments (air, surface water, subsurface water, and soil) and technical compartments (production, manufacturing, consumption, sewage treatment plants, waste incineration plants, landfills, reprocessing, elimination, and export). Based on global market size estimates and projected growth rates for NCMs, the production growth rate and market share within the European Union were determined. Because validated transfer coefficients specific to NCMs were not available, values were adopted from studies on other engineered nanomaterials. To account for the substantial uncertainty associated with these assumptions, Bayesian estimation techniques were applied to propagate uncertainties and estimate plausible environmental concentration ranges for NCMs. PEC distributions were generated using Monte Carlo simulations based on the assigned parameter distributions. All analyses were conducted using the dpmfa-simulator (https://pypi.org/project/dpmfa-simulator/). The analysis predicted that the average annual production volume of NCMs in the EU would increase from approximately 1405 tons in 2005 to 30,603 tons by 2025. Among environmental compartments, soil received the highest estimated inflow, while surface water received the lowest, with an average annual inflow of approximately 150 tons across the EU.

8.3.2 Calculation of PNEC

The PNEC for surface water was calculated as a probability distribution using Monte Carlo simulations, following the methodology described by Coll et al. (2016) and Wigger et al. (2020). When ecotoxicity data are limited in a small number of species, constructing a PSSD enables appropriate reflection of data uncertainty in the PNEC estimation.

To calculate PNEC, effect concentrations such as the 50% effective concentration (EC_{50}) for individual species were first collected. Only in vivo tests (ecotoxicity studies using whole organisms—investigating NCM effects on survival, growth, or reproduction in freshwater, air, or soil) were considered. Rather than relying on a

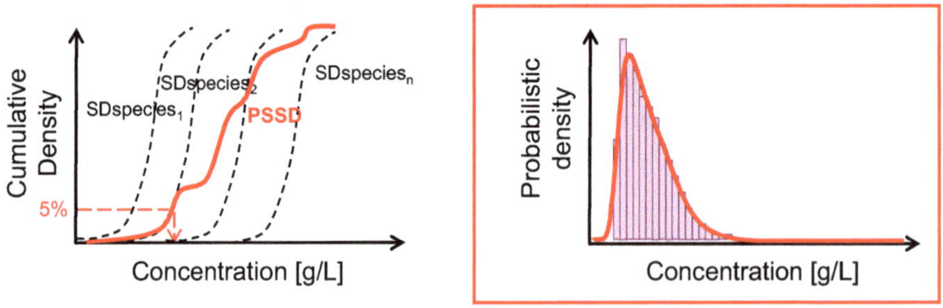

Fig. 8.2 Conceptual diagram modeling PSSD for a specific environmental compartment PSSD is generated by synthesizing Monte Carlo simulation results for species-specific SSDs. PNEC is derived from the 5th percentile of PSSD, resulting in a probabilistic PNEC distribution. The red box illustrates the conceptual diagram of the PNEC distribution using the 5th percentile value of PSSD

single toxicity endpoint per species, all available endpoints were expressed as probability density functions to construct species-specific sensitivity distributions. A conceptual diagram is shown in Fig. 8.2. The endpoints obtained for each species were converted to chronic NOECs using two assessment factors accounting for exposure duration and dose–response relationships. The 5th percentile value of the synthesized sensitivity distribution for the entire surface water compartment was defined as the PNEC, in accordance with the guidelines of the European Chemicals Agency (ECHA).

Based on the literature review, ecotoxicity data from five studies meeting the PSSD criteria were included (Harper et al. 2016; Kovacs et al. 2010; Ogonowski et al. 2018; Ong et al. 2017; Wang et al. 2020). These studies encompassed 8 species and 76 toxicity endpoints, all relevant to surface water exposure (Table 8.1). Using these data, a PSSD was constructed. Based on the 5th percentile value of this PSSD, the mean PNEC was 7.69 mg/L and the mode was 2.11 mg/L.

8.3.3 Risk Characterization

The PEC distributions for 2015 and 2025 were calculated based on the estimated mass of NCMs present in surface waters for each year, obtained through DPMFA. Environmental concentrations were derived by dividing the estimated mass of NCMs in the surface water compartment by the total volume of surface water within the European Union.

Using the resulting PEC and PNEC probability distributions, RCR was calculated. For 2015, the overlap between the PEC and PNEC distributions was minimal, and the mean RCR was estimated to be 6.9×10^{-5}, indicating negligible ecological risk at that time. For 2025, the mean RCR increased to 7.1×10^{-4}. Compared with 2015, the increased discharge in 2025 caused the peak of the PEC distribution to approach the PNEC distribution, resulting in a modest increase in RCR. Nevertheless, even under the 2025 scenario, the degree of overlap between PEC and PNEC distributions remained extremely small, indicating that the ecological risk of NCMs to aquatic organisms in surface waters is expected to remain very low.

Although these results are based on data from the European Union, similar conclusions are anticipated for Japan. While the assessment is based on a limited ecotoxicity dataset, the accumulation of additional ecotoxicity data in the future will allow for more reliable risk estimations.

8.4 Key Findings from the NEDO Project

8.4.1 Overview of the Initiative

The NEDO project (FY2020–2024) placed a strong emphasis on ecological impact assessment, defined as the quantification of adverse effects on organisms or biological communities within ecological risk assessment frameworks. The primary objective was to derive ecologically relevant impact assessment values for CNFs with respect to freshwater aquatic organisms. This section provides an overview of the initiative.

When CNFs are released into the environment, their exposure potential to aquatic organisms is strongly influenced by the water quality of the receiving environment (Tai et al. 2022). For example, divalent cations such as calcium and magnesium commonly present in natural waters can promote CNF agglomeration and sedimentation, thereby reducing the exposure potential to aquatic organisms. Consequently, detailed ecological impact assessments of CNFs are required for each water environment with different water quality conditions. However, such comprehensive testing requires substantial time and resources. To establish a practical and reproducible baseline, the NEDO project conducted ecotoxicity tests under controlled conditions in which CNF properties remained relatively stable due to the water quality of the test medium, and CNF dispersion was maintained throughout the exposure period. The resulting data provide foundational knowledge for future ecological impact and risk assessments of CNFs under specific environmental conditions.

Tai et al. (2022) reviewed existing literature on CNF ecotoxicity tests and identified several key considerations for conducting such tests. Several studies suggested that differences in CNF manufacturing methods could lead to varying ecological effects on aquatic organisms. In addition, many studies lacked adequate characterization of CNF exposure, particularly with respect to agglomeration and sedimentation. Based on these studies and the OECD guidance document 317 on the ecotoxicity testing of nanomaterials, it was therefore considered essential to verify whether CNFs remain stably dispersed in the test media throughout the exposure period. Additional CNF-specific considerations include uptake by test organisms (e.g., reduced feeding activity and consequent decreases in CNF concentrations), nutrient depletion due to adsorption onto CNFs, interference of CNFs with algal biomass measurements, interference from test organisms (mainly algae) or feed (mainly *Chlorella* spp. used for *D. magna* feeding) in CNF concentration analysis, and the influence of microorganisms (fungi, bacteria) or preservatives. Addressing these factors is essential for conducting appropriate ecotoxicity tests for CNFs, and test methods should be optimized for each CNF type.

Figure 8.3 illustrates the research flow adopted for ecological impact assessment in the NEDO project. First, two analytical methods were developed to accurately quantify CNF concentrations while minimizing interference from test organisms or feed. Subsequently, for each target CNF type, short-term (acute) and medium-to-long-term (subchronic and chronic) ecotoxicity tests were conducted using algae, *Daphnia* species, and fish, following the establishment of suitable test conditions. For CNFs prone to sedimentation and unsuitable for medium-to-longer-term *D. magna* exposure tests, ecotoxicity assessments were performed using benthic amphipods.

The types of ecotoxicity tests conducted in the project are summarized in Table 8.3. Based on the resulting ecotoxicity values, PNECs were derived as ecological impact assessment values for CNFs. Four CNF types produced via different manufacturing methods were evaluated: TEMPO-oxidized CNFs, mechanically

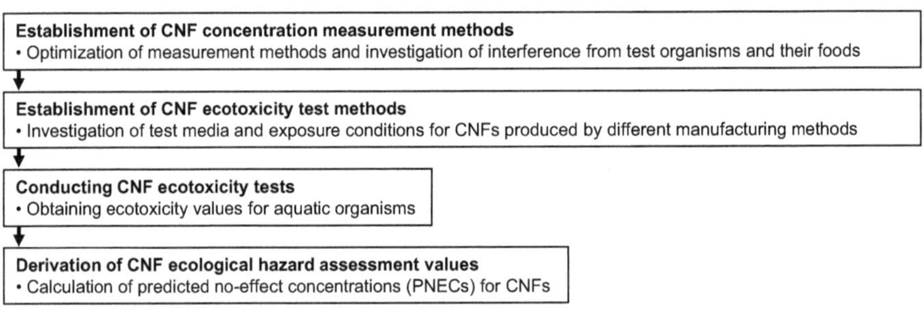

Fig. 8.3 Research flow of ecological impact assessment

Table 8.3 Ecotoxicity tests conducted in the NEDO project

Ecotoxicity test	OECD TG No.	Toxicity type	Test organism	Measured endpoint
Algal growth inhibition test	201[a]	Acute/ chronic	*Raphidocelis subcapitata*	Growth rate
Daphnia sp. immobilisation test	202[b]	Acute	*Daphnia magna*	Swimming behavior
Fish acute toxicity test	203[c]	Acute	*Oryzias latipes* (Medaka)	Survival
Daphnia magna reproduction test	211[d]	Chronic	*Daphnia magna*	Cumulative offspring count
Amphipod subchronic toxicity test	–[e]	Subchronic	*Amphipod*	Survival and growth
Fish early life stage toxicity test	210[f]	Chronic	*Oryzias latipes* (Medaka)	Survival

Notes: [a]OECD (2011), [b]OECD (2004), [c]OECD (2025a), [d]OECD (2012), [e]No OECD TG available, referenced U.S. EPA (2000), [f]OECD (2025b)

fibrillated CNFs produced by the aqueous counter collision method, mechanically fibrillated CNFs produced by the water-jet method, and phosphorylated CNFs. The following sections outline the results obtained at each stage of the research workflow.

8.4.2 Establishment of CNF Concentration Measurement Methods

Because CNFs readily agglomerate and sediment in aqueous media, verification of their concentration and dispersion state in test solutions is essential for the appropriate conduct and interpretation of ecotoxicity tests. However, existing reports lack established methods for quantifying CNF concentrations. To address this gap, two analytical methods that are simple, cost-effective, and suitable for high-throughput analysis were developed and validated to quantify CNFs in the test solutions (Fig. 8.4).

The first method is a modified version of the phenol-sulfuric acid method, commonly used for sugar analysis, adapted for use with microplates. In this approach, CNFs are decomposed by sulfuric acid and subsequently react with phenol to produce a colorimetric response that is quantified by spectrophotometric absorbance measurement. The use of microplates substantially reduces reagent consumption and enables simultaneous analysis of multiple samples. Unlike the conventional tube-based method, which relies on heat generated by the addition of sulfuric acid, the microplate method requires external heating (~90 °C) using a thermal mixer due to the smaller reaction volume and reduced heat generation. In addition, whereas the conventional protocol adds phenol prior to sulfuric acid addition, it was found that adding phenol after sulfuric acid heating enhances color development. Although this method quantifies total sugars and does not selectively quantify cellulose, it is

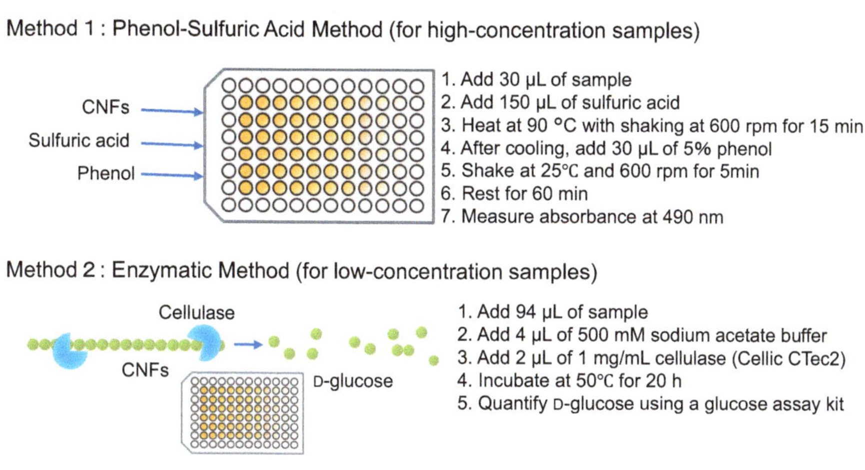

Fig. 8.4 Analytical methods for CNF quantification in ecotoxicity testing

well suited for ecotoxicity test solutions in which other sugars are largely absent, allowing reliable quantification of added CNFs. Detailed methodological information is provided in Ogura et al. (2023).

The second method involves enzymatic hydrolysis of CNFs into glucose using cellulase, followed by glucose quantification with a commercial glucose assay kit and spectrophotometric analysis. Because commercial cellulase contains impurities such as glucose, the enzyme was purified prior to use. Among the three cellulase types tested, Merck's Cellic CTec2 exhibited the highest efficiency for CNF degradation. This method selectively quantifies cellulose and is less susceptible to interference from noncellulosic components in test solutions. Further details are described in Ogura et al. (2020) and Matsuzawa et al. (2024).

Test solutions for ecotoxicity studies typically contain culture medium components, test organisms, feed, and metabolic waste products. Both analytical methods were confirmed to be applicable for quantifying mechanically fibrillated CNFs, TEMPO-oxidized CNFs, and phosphorylated CNFs in such complex matrices. However, algae used in algal growth inhibition tests contain cellulose as a structural component, and algal biomass accumulation over the 72-h exposure period can interfere with CNF quantification. Accordingly, corrections such as subtraction of algal-derived cellulose contributions are required (Sect. 8.4.3.4). Notably, the enzymatic method exhibited lower susceptibility to algal interference. Interference from *C. vulgaris*, which is used as feed in *Daphnia* tests, was negligible with respect to CNF concentration measurements.

Both methods rely solely on spectrophotometric measurements using a microplate reader and do not require specialized or expensive analytical instrumentation. The phenol–sulfuric acid method involves hazardous reagents, including phenol and sulfuric acid, whereas the glucose assay kit used in the enzymatic method is relatively expensive. The detection limit of the phenol–sulfuric acid method is approximately 10 mg/L, while the enzymatic method achieves detection limits below 1 mg/L. Thus, the phenol–sulfuric acid method offers simplicity and cost efficiency, whereas the enzymatic method provides higher sensitivity and reduced susceptibility to matrix interference. Selection of the appropriate method should therefore be based on the CNF concentration range and sample complexity. In the NEDO ecotoxicity studies, CNF concentrations of 12.5 mg/L or lower were quantified using the enzymatic method, whereas concentrations of 25–100 mg/L were measured using the phenol–sulfuric acid method. Both analytical approaches are applicable not only to CNFs but also to general cellulose analysis.

8.4.3 Establishment of Ecotoxicity Testing Methods for CNFs

8.4.3.1 Selection of Test Media and Evaluation of CNF Dispersion Stability

Nutrient salts in the test medium are essential for the growth of aquatic organisms. However, higher ion concentrations tend to promote agglomeration and sedimentation of CNFs. From the perspective of maintaining CNF dispersion stability, test media with lower ion concentrations are therefore preferable. For ecotoxicity tests using *D. magna* and *Oryzias latipes* (medaka), test media with sufficiently low ion concentrations that do not affect growth, survival, or reproduction were selected, and the dispersion stability of each CNF type was evaluated.

As an example, Fig. 8.5 presents the dispersion stability evaluation results for TEMPO-oxidized CNFs in media with different ionic compositions. A comparison was made between "moderate-hardness synthetic water," a standard medium published by the U.S. Environmental Protection Agency (U.S. EPA 2002), and a lower-ionic-strength medium prepared by blending "low-hardness synthetic water" (also published by the U.S. EPA) with dechlorinated tap water at an 8:2 ratio. TEMPO-oxidized CNFs remained stably dispersed in the 8:2 blended medium, and this formulation was therefore adopted for subsequent testing (Tai et al. 2024a). For phosphorylated CNFs, dispersion stability in the 8:2 blended medium was slightly reduced; consequently, a 9:1 blended water was used instead.

For mechanically fibrillated CNFs, the 9:1 blended water was also used. However, sedimentation of CNFs was observed under static conditions. To improve dispersion stability without affecting organism survival, gentle agitation was applied during testing. Specifically, horizontal shaking at 100 rpm was used in the *D. magna* immobilisation test, and magnetic stirring at 150 rpm was applied in the medaka acute toxicity test.

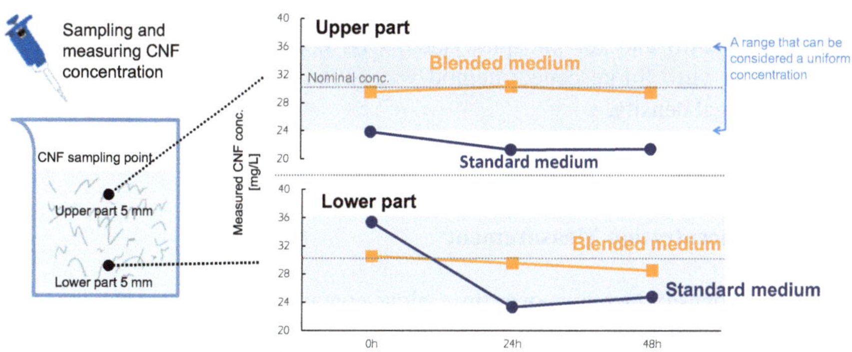

Fig. 8.5 Evaluation of test media and concentration uniformity for TEMPO-oxidized CNFs. The target CNF concentration was 30 mg/L. A concentration range within ±20% of the target value was considered acceptable

For the algal growth inhibition test, the composition of the test medium and agitation conditions are specified in OECD TG 201, and the test was conducted in accordance with this guideline (OECD 2011).

8.4.3.2 Reduction of Nutrient Salts Due to Adsorption onto CNFs

For TEMPO-oxidized CNFs, a reduction in nutrient salt concentrations in the test medium was observed, attributable to adsorption of ions onto CNFs (Tai et al. 2024a, b). Similarly, phosphorylated CNFs also caused a reduction in nutrient salt concentrations. Despite these changes, no adverse effects on algal growth or organism survival were detected. In contrast, mechanically fibrillated CNFs did not cause measurable reductions in nutrient salt concentrations under the tested conditions.

8.4.3.3 Interference of CNFs with Algal Biomass Measurement in Algal Tests

In algal growth inhibition tests, growth rates are typically calculated based on changes in algal density over the exposure period. However, the presence of CNFs in the dispersions may interfere with algal density measurements. In particular, particle counters commonly used for cell counting can mistakenly count CNF particles as algal cells. To address this issue, two fluorescence-based methods were employed to quantify algal biomass using chlorophyll content as a proxy: (i) in vivo fluorescence measurement, which directly measures chlorophyll fluorescence in living algal cells, and (ii) in vitro fluorescence measurement, which quantifies chlorophyll fluorescence in solvent extracts of the test solution. The potential interference of CNFs with these measurements was evaluated. The results confirmed that both methods were suitable for TEMPO-oxidized CNFs (Tai et al. 2024b) and for phosphorylated CNFs. For mechanically fibrillated CNFs, the in vitro fluorescence method was found to be more appropriate for measuring algal density.

8.4.3.4 Interference of Test Organisms and Feed with CNF Concentration Measurement

As algal cell density increases over time, algae containing cellulose—can interfere with CNF quantification. In fact, algae grown for 72 h after test initiation were found to slightly affect CNF quantification. This interference was corrected by subtracting the algal-derived contribution from the measured CNF concentrations (Tai et al. 2024b). Specifically, algal density and the corresponding CNF-equivalent concentration were first measured in the control group. The CNF-equivalent concentration per algal cell was then calculated by dividing the CNF-equivalent concentration by algal density. This value was then multiplied by the algal density measured in each exposure group after 72 h to estimate the algal-derived CNF-equivalent concentration, which was subsequently subtracted from the measured CNF concentration for each group. Figure 8.6 shows the interference caused by algae in CNF concentration measurements during the algal growth inhibition tests using TEMPO-oxidized CNFs, as well as the corrected CNF concentrations after subtracting the algal-derived CNFs. Similar corrections were applied to other CNF types. In contrast, *C. vulgaris*, which was used as feed in the *D. magna* reproduction test, did not interfere with CNF measurements (Matsuzawa et al. 2024).

8.4.3.5 Consideration of Effects from Fungi, Bacteria, and Preservatives

To prevent the proliferation of fungi and bacteria on CNFs during ecotoxicity testing, appropriate sterilization methods were evaluated. It was confirmed that 2-phenoxyethanol, a preservative commonly used in pharmaceutical formulations, adversely affected *D. magna* at concentrations required for effective sterilization (Mano 2021). Conversely, gamma irradiation at an absorbed dose of 1 kGy was found to effectively sterilize CNFs while inducing only minimal changes in their morphology and physicochemical properties (Horie et al. 2023; Ogura et al. 2025). Based on these findings, all CNF materials used in the ecotoxicity tests were sterilized by exposure to 1 kGy gamma radiation.

8.4.4 Results of Ecotoxicity Tests on CNFs

The results of ecotoxicity tests conducted under the NEDO project for four types of CNFs—TEMPO-oxidized CNFs, mechanically fibrillated CNFs (aqueous counter collision method), mechanically fibrillated CNFs (water-jet method), and phosphorylated CNFs—are summarized in Table 8.4. Values in boldface indicate the lowest toxicity value observed for each CNF type. Test CNF concentrations were generally set at 0, 3.1, 6.3, 12.5, 25, 50, and 100 mg/L. In most tests, no adverse effects were observed even at the highest concentration of 100 mg/L (EC_{50}, LC_{50} > 100 mg/L; NOEC ≥ 100 mg/L). However, in the *D. magna* reproduction test using TEMPO-oxidized CNFs, a significant reduction in cumulative offspring count was observed at concentrations of 25 mg/L and above, resulting in a calculated NOEC of 12.5 mg/L. This reproductive effect is thought to be due to *D. magna* ingesting CNFs through filter feeding at high concentrations, which reduced the intake of *C. vulgaris*—the primary food source—thereby impairing growth and reproduction (Mano et al. 2025). Supporting this interpretation, when *D.* magna neonates were exposed to 100 mg/L CNFs for 24 h and then transferred to CNF-free medium containing *C. vulgaris*, the CNFs present in their gut were excreted within 24 h. This finding suggests that continuous exposure to high CNF concentrations is required for reproductive effects to manifest.

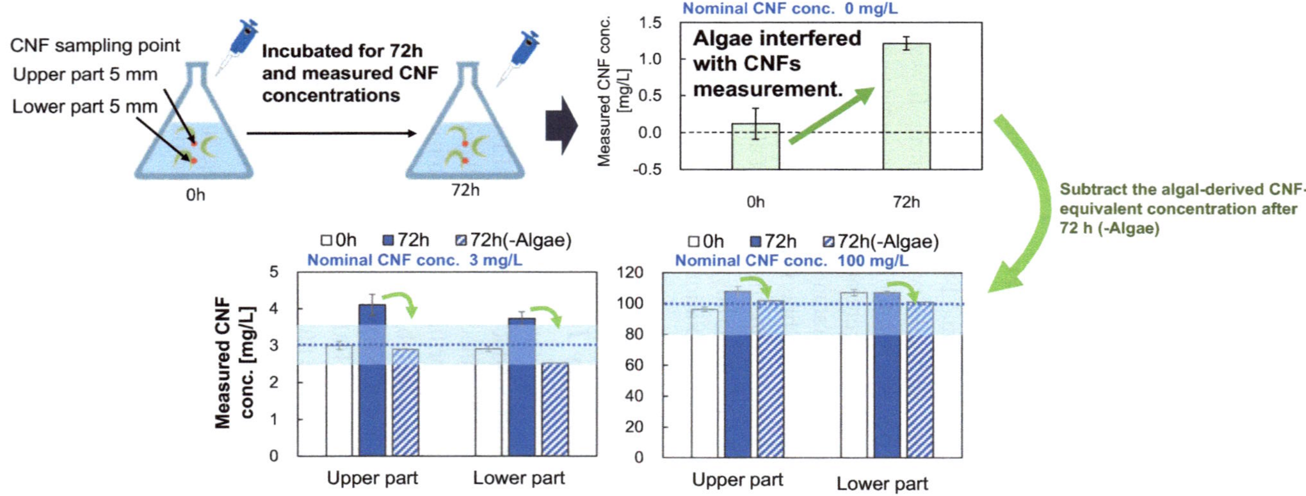

Fig. 8.6 Algal interference in CNF concentration measurements and correction in the algal growth inhibition test for TEMPO-oxidized CNFs
CNF concentrations were measured at the start of the test (0 h) and after 72 h of cultivation (72 h). "72 h (-Algae)" indicates the CNF concentration after subtracting the CNF-equivalent concentration derived from algae

Table 8.4 CNF ecotoxicity values obtained in the NEDO project

Ecotoxicity test	Toxicity	TEMPO--oxidized CNFs	Mechanically fibrillated CNFs (ACC)	Mechanically fibrillated CNFs (WJ)	Phosphorylated CNFs
Algal growth inhibition test (acute)	EC_{50}	>100 mg/L[a]	>100 mg/L	>100 mg/L	Under analysis
Algal growth inhibition test (chronic)	NOEC	≥100 mg/L[a]	**≥100 mg/L**	**≥100 mg/L**	Under analysis
Daphnia sp. immobilisation test (acute)	EC_{50}	>100 mg/L[b]	>100 mg/L	>100 mg/L	**>100 mg/L**
Fish acute toxicity test (acute)	LC_{50}	>100 mg/L[b]	>100 mg/L	>100 mg/L	**>100 mg/L**
Daphnia magna reproduction test (chronic)	NOEC	**12.5 mg/L**[c]	–	–	Under analysis
Amphipod subchronic toxicity test (subchronic)	NOEC	–	–	Under analysis	–
Fish early life stage toxicity test (chronic)	NOEC	≥100 mg/L	–	–	–

Bolded toxicity values indicate the lowest toxicity value for each CNF type
ACC Aqueous counter collision method, *WJ* water-jet method
[a]Tai et al. (2024b), [b]Tai et al. (2024a), [c]Mano et al. (2025)

Although reproduction test results for other CNF types are not yet available, similar effects have been reported for mechanically fibrillated CNFs, where reduced offspring production was observed at 20.6 mg/L and significantly decreased feeding rates were detected at concentrations of 10–20 mg/L (Ogonowski et al. 2018). These findings suggest that the observed reproductive effects are not specific to a particular CNF type. Furthermore, reduced feeding rates in *D. magna* have also been observed upon exposure to polystyrene particles (1 mg/L; 100 nm or 2 μm) (Rist et al. 2017), indicating that this phenomenon is not unique to CNFs.

For contextual interpretation, the ecotoxicity values obtained from the tests were evaluated using the toxicity rating tables published in the 2019 report by Group of Experts on the Scientific Aspects of Marine Environmental Protection (GESAMP), organized by the United Nations. Table 8.5 shows the acute toxicity rating scale from GESAMP (2019), and the acute toxicity values for CNFs listed in Table 8.4 fall under Rating 1: "Practically nontoxic." Similarly, according to the chronic toxicity rating scale shown in Table 8.6, the chronic toxicity values for CNFs fall under Rating 0: "Negligible,"Overall, the acute and chronic toxicity data generated in this NEDO project indicate that the CNF types tested exhibit low ecotoxicity toward aquatic organisms under the tested conditions.

Table 8.5 Ratings for acute toxicity (GESAMP 2019)

Rating	Description	Toxicity value (EC_{50}, LC_{50}) [mg/L]
0	Nontoxic	>1000
1	Practically nontoxic	>100 and ≤1000
2	Slightly toxic	>10 and ≤100
3	Moderately toxic	>1 and ≤10
4	Highly toxic	>0.1 and ≤1
5	Very highly toxic	>0.01 and ≤0.1
6	Extremely toxic	≤0.01

Table 8.6 Ratings for chronic toxicity (GESAMP 2019)

Rating	Description	Toxicity value (NOEC) [mg/L]
0	Negligible	>1
1	Low	>0.1 and ≤1
2	Moderate	>0.01 and ≤0.1
3	High	>0.001 and ≤0.01
4	Very high	≤0.001

8.4.5 Derivation of PNEC

To enable businesses handling CNFs to voluntarily predict and assess the ecological risks associated with environmental release from their facilities, it is necessary to establish ecological impact assessment values—specifically, the PNEC—that can be compared with estimated environmental discharge volumes based on planned production and other operational data. Accordingly, PNEC values were derived using the results obtained in the NEDO project, with reference to the risk assessment of priority assessment chemical substances under Japan's Chemical Substances Control Law (CSCL) (Ministry of Health, Labour and Welfare; Ministry of Economy, Trade and Industry; Ministry of the Environment 2014). For each of the four CNF types evaluated—TEMPO-oxidized CNFs, mechanically fibrillated CNFs (aqueous counter collision method), mechanically fibrillated CNFs (water-jet method), and phosphorylated CNFs—the lowest available toxicity value was divided by a total uncertainty factor, determined according to the extent of available data, to calculate PNEC.

Because toxicity values obtained from laboratory tests using test organisms are extrapolated to predict effects on organisms in natural environments, and various uncertainties arise from factors such as test duration, it is necessary to consider appropriate uncertainty factors (UFs). UFs and their total used for deriving PNECs for aquatic organisms, as specified in the CSCL guidance, are summarized in Table 8.7. The total UF depends on the extent of available ecotoxicity data. Based on the data coverage presented in Table 8.4, the total UF was set to 10 for TEMPO-oxidized CNFs and 100 for mechanically fibrillated CNFs. For phosphorylated CNFs, the total UF varied depending on the species used for toxicity evaluation:

Table 8.7 Factors of uncertainty and uncertainty factor (UF) values[a]

Toxicity value used	UF for interspecies extrapolation	UF for acute to chronic extrapolation	UF for laboratory to field extrapolation	Total UF
Lowest chronic toxicity value from three trophic levels	–	–	10	10
Lower chronic toxicity value from two trophic levels	5	–	10	50
NOEC from one trophic level chronic toxicity test	10	–	10	100
Lowest acute toxicity value from three trophic levels	–	ACR[b]	10	10 × ACR
Lower acute toxicity value when chronic data are missing for some trophic levels	10	ACR	10	100 × ACR

Notes: [a]Adapted from Figure III-4 of the Risk Assessment Guidance for Priority Assessment Chemical Substances under the Chemical Substances Control Law (MHLW, METI, MOE 2014), [b]ACR: Acute-to-Chronic Ratio—20 for algae, 10 for daphnids, 100 for fish

1000 when using *D. magna* toxicity data and 10,000 when using fish toxicity data. To ensure a conservative assessment of ecological impact, the higher UF value of 10,000 was adopted.

Using these UFs, the PNEC values were calculated by dividing the lowest toxicity value (from Table 8.4) by the total UF as follows:

- TEMPO-oxidized CNFs: 1.25 mg/L (12.5 mg/L ÷ 10)
- Mechanically fibrillated CNFs: ≥1 mg/L (≥100 mg/L ÷ 100)
- Phosphorylated CNFs: >0.01 mg/L (>100 mg/L ÷ 10,000)

It should be noted that the PNEC for phosphorylated CNFs was derived from only two acute toxicity values. Consequently, the large total UF substantially influences PNEC due to the limited ecotoxicity data currently available. Therefore, it is necessary to re-calculate PNEC once the ongoing ecotoxicity data analyses are completed.

When applying the PNEC values of the three CNF types to the ecological hazard classification framework used in CSCL screening evaluations—which consists of five categories (Class 1 to Class 4 and "Outside Class")—TEMPO-oxidized CNFs and mechanically fibrillated CNFs were classified as "Outside Class." Phosphorylated CNFs were classified as Class 3. Under CSCL screening criteria, chemical substances classified as Class 3 are not considered to pose ecological risks provided that their total domestic discharge does not exceed 1000 tons, and therefore do not require further detailed ecological risk assessment.

8.5 Summary

8.5.1 Findings from Existing Literature

In existing reports on CNFs, two studies have documented effects on algae even at the lowest test concentration of 1 mg/L (Pereira et al. 2014; Munk et al. 2015). Pereira et al. (2014) suggested that gum-like cellulose structures formed around algal cells increased CNF adsorption to the algal cell surface, interfering with gas exchange at the cell wall and nutrient uptake at the cell membrane, thereby inhibiting the growth of *C. vulgaris*. In contrast, other studies reported no observable effects on algae even at substantially higher concentrations (Wang et al. 2020; Ong et al. 2017).

In acute toxicity tests using *D. magna*, slight immobilization has been reported at concentrations of 20–40 mg/L (Kokol et al. 2023; Vartiainen et al. 2011), whereas several other studies observed no effects even at the highest test concentrations evaluated (Wang et al. 2020; Pengiran et al. 2022; Ogonowski et al. 2018; Ong et al. 2017). Only one study has reported chronic toxicity data for *D. magna*, showing reduced offspring production at 20.6 mg/L and a significant decrease in feeding rates at concentrations of 10–20 mg/L (Ogonowski et al. 2018). In acute toxicity tests using zebrafish, one study reported a significant increase in mortality and elevated incidence of yolk sac and pericardial edema at 250 mg/L (Harper et al. 2016). However, many other studies reported no observable effects even at the highest concentrations tested (Wang et al. 2020; Pengiran et al. 2022; Harper et al. 2016; Ong et al. 2017; Liu et al. 2020). Overall, the available literature suggests that the impact of CNFs on aquatic organisms—including algae, crustaceans, and fish—is relatively low compared to general chemical substances.

8.5.2 Insights from the NEDO Project

Previous ecotoxicity studies have often lacked sufficient evaluation of CNF exposure conditions—particularly with respect to CNF concentration and dispersion state in the test medium—raising concerns about the validity and comparability of test outcomes. To address these limitations, the NEDO project first established reliable methods for quantifying CNF concentrations and then developed ecotoxicity testing protocols tailored to each CNF type. In developing these protocols, key factors influencing test reliability were systematically addressed, including CNF dispersion stability, uptake by test organisms (e.g., reduced feeding rates, decreased CNF concentration), nutrient depletion resulting from adsorption onto CNFs, interference of CNFs with algal biomass measurements, interference of test organisms (primarily algae) and food sources (mainly *Chlorella* spp. used for *D. magna*) with CNF concentration measurements, and potential effects of fungi, bacteria, and preservatives.

Ecotoxicity tests were conducted on four types of CNFs: TEMPO-oxidized CNFs, mechanically fibrillated CNFs (aqueous counter collision method), mechanically fibrillated CNFs (water-jet method), and phosphorylated CNFs. The test battery included algal growth inhibition tests, *D. magna* immobilisation tests, and fish acute toxicity tests. In addition, *D. magna* reproduction tests were performed for two CNF types, while fish early-life-stage toxicity tests and amphipod subchronic toxicity tests were each conducted for one CNF type. In most tests, no adverse effects were observed even at the highest test concentration of 100 mg/L. However, in the *D. magna* reproduction test using TEMPO-oxidized CNFs, a significant reduction in cumulative offspring count was observed at concentrations ≥25 mg/L. This effect was attributed to *D. magna* ingesting CNFs via filter feeding, which reduced food intake and consequently impaired growth and reproduction. Although reproduction test results for CNF types other than TEMPO-oxidized CNFs are not yet available, similar findings have been reported for mechanically fibrillated CNFs (Ogonowski et al. 2018), suggesting that this phenomenon may not be specific to a particular CNF type. Moreover, reduced feeding rates in *Daphnia* have also been reported for polystyrene particles (Rist et al. 2017), indicating that this response is not unique to CNFs. Based on the magnitude of the observed toxicity values, CNFs are considered to exhibit relatively low ecotoxicity compared with general chemical substances.

Ecological impact assessment values, i.e., PNECs, were derived to provide benchmarks for CNF management. For each CNF type, the lowest available toxicity value was divided by a total UF reflecting the extent of available ecotoxicity data. For TEMPO-oxidized CNFs, with available chronic toxicity data for three trophic levels, PNEC was calculated as 1.25 mg/L (12.5 mg/L ÷ UF 10). For mechanically fibrillated CNFs, for which chronic toxicity data are available for one trophic level and acute toxicity data for the other two, PNEC was ≥1 mg/L (≥100 mg/L ÷ UF 100). For phosphorylated CNFs, with available acute toxicity data for only two trophic levels, PNEC was calculated as >0.01 mg/L (>100 mg/L ÷ UF 10,000). However, given the limited ecotoxicity dataset for phosphorylated CNFs and the resulting high UF, further data acquisition is necessary to reassess its ecological impact.

8.5.3 Future Challenges

In some algal studies, effects were reported even at the lowest test concentration of 1 mg/L. Further data accumulation is therefore needed to clarify differences in algal responses depending on CNF type. Similarly, chronic toxicity data for *Daphnia* species and fish remain limited, and additional data collection is necessary.

Given that CNFs tend to agglomerate and settle in the presence of ions such as calcium and magnesium commonly found in environmental water, it is likely that CNFs accumulate in sediments. Accordingly, ecotoxicity data for benthic organisms should be expanded in addition to studies on algae, crustaceans, and fish.

Within the NEDO project, robust methods for CNF quantification were established, and test conditions suitable for CNFs were developed by explicitly considering factors such as dispersion stability (Sects. 8.4.2 and 8.4.3). It is anticipated that these findings will serve as a valuable reference for businesses designing future ecotoxicity testing protocols for NCMs.

References

Blaise C, Vasseur P (2005) Algal microplate toxicity test. In: Blaise C, Férard JF (eds) Small-scale freshwater toxicity investigations, vol 1. Springer, Dordrecht, pp 137–179. https://doi.org/10.1007/1-4020-3120-3_4

Coll C, Notter D, Gottschalk F, Sun T, Som C, Nowack B (2016) Probabilistic environmental risk assessment of five nanomaterials (nano-TiO2, nano-Ag, nano-ZnO, CNT, and fullerenes). Nanotoxicology 10(4):436–444. https://doi.org/10.3109/17435390.2015.1073812

Environment Canada (2000a) Biological test method: reference method for determining acute lethality of effluent to rainbow trout. EPS 1/RM/13, 2nd edn

Environment Canada (2000b) Biological test method: reference method for determining acute lethality of effluent to *Daphnia magna*. EPS 1/RM/14, 2nd edn

Environment Canada (2007) Biological test method: test of reproduction and survival using the Cladoceran *Ceriodaphnia dubia*. EPS 1/RM/21, 2nd edn

Esposito MC, Riva L, Russo GL, Punta C, Corsi I, Tosti E, Gallo A (2024) Reproductive toxicity assessment of cellulose nanofibers, citric acid, and branched polyethylenimine in sea urchins: eco-design of nanostructured cellulose sponge framework (Part B). Environ Pollut 350:12. https://doi.org/10.1016/j.envpol.2024.123934

GESAMP (2019) GESAMP hazard evaluation procedure for chemicals carried by ships, 2019. Joint group of experts on the scientific aspects of marine environmental protection, Rep. Stud. GESAMP No. 102. http://www.gesamp.org/site/assets/files/2133/rs102e.pdf. Accessed 28 Nov 2024

Harper BJ, Clendaniel A, Sinche F, Way D, Hughes M, Schardt J, Simonsen J, Stefaniak AB, Harper SL (2016) Impacts of chemical modification on the toxicity of diverse nanocellulose materials to developing zebrafish. Cellulose (London, England) 23(3):1763–1775. https://doi.org/10.1007/s10570-016-0947-5

Hill AJ, Teraoka H, Heideman W, Peterson RE (2005) Zebrafish as a model vertebrate for investigating chemical toxicity. Toxicol Sci 86(1):6–19. https://doi.org/10.1093/toxsci/kfi110

Horie M, Fujita K, Endoh S, Sugino S, Maru J, Moriyama A, Ogura I (2023) Contaminant microorganisms in the *in vitro* evaluation of cellular responses of cellulose nanofibers and their microbial inactivation using gamma irradiation. Toxicol Mech Methods 33(9):741–754. https://doi.org/10.1080/15376516.2023.2238061

ISO (2011) ISO 14380:2011, Water quality—determination of the acute toxicity to *Thamnocephalus platyurus* (Crustacea, Anostraca)

Kokol V, Novak S, Kononenko V, Kos M, Vivod V, Gunde-Cimerman N, Drobne D (2023) Antibacterial and degradation properties of dialdehyded and aminohexamethylated nanocelluloses. Carbohydr Polym 311:120603. https://doi.org/10.1016/j.carbpol.2023.120603

Kovacs T, Martel P, Ricci M (2007) A short-term adult fathead minnow reproduction test for investigation of cause and investigation of solution work involving pulp and paper mill effluents. Water Qual Res J Can 42:91–100

Kovacs T, Naish V, O'Connor B, Blaise C, Gagné F, Hall L, Trudeau V, Martel P (2010) An ecotoxicological characterization of nanocrystalline cellulose (NCC). Nanotoxicology 4(3):255–270. https://doi.org/10.3109/17435391003628713

Liu C, Zhao J, Zhang X, Wei G, Hao W, Wang X, Yang C, Shi Y, Liu D (2020) Biomass-derived cellulose nanoparticles display considerable neurotoxicity in zebrafish. Int J Biol Macromol 165(B):1783–1792. https://doi.org/10.1016/j.ijbiomac.2020.10.033

Mano H (2021) Chronic toxicity of 2-phenoxyethanol to *Daphnia magna*. Jpn J Environ Toxicol 24:48–52

Mano H, Tai R, Moriyama A, Iizumi Y, Matsuzawa T, Okazaki T, Ogura I (2025) Dilution effect of TEMPO-oxidized cellulose nanofibers on reproduction of *Daphnia magna*. Ecotoxicol Environ Saf 294:11. https://doi.org/10.1016/j.ecoenv.2025.118101

Matsuzawa T, Tai R, Mano H, Ogura I (2024) Applicability of enzymatic and phenol-sulfuric acid methods for determination of cellulose nanofibers in ecotoxicity testing. J Wood Sci 70(1):17. https://doi.org/10.1186/s10086-024-02131-7

Ministry of Health, Labour and Welfare, Ministry of Economy, Trade and Industry, Ministry of the Environment (2014) Technical guidance for risk assessment of priority assessment chemical substances under the Chemical Substances Control Law. https://www.meti.go.jp/policy/chemical_management/kasinhou/files/information/ra/tech_guidance_full_202207.pdf (in Japanese)

Munk M, Brandão HM, Nowak S, Mouton L, Gern JC, Guimaraes AS, Yéprémian C, Couté A, Raposo NRB, Marconcini JM, Brayner R (2015) Direct and indirect toxic effects of cotton--derived cellulose nanofibres on filamentous green algae. Ecotoxicol Environ Saf 122:399–405. https://doi.org/10.1016/j.ecoenv.2015.09.001

OECD (2004) Test no. 202: *Daphnia* sp. acute immobilisation test, OECD guidelines for the testing of chemicals, section 2. OECD Publishing, Paris. https://doi.org/10.1787/9789264069947-en

OECD (2011) Test no. 201: freshwater alga and cyanobacteria, growth inhibition test, OECD guidelines for the testing of chemicals, section 2. OECD Publishing, Paris. https://doi.org/10.1787/9789264069923-en

OECD (2012) Test no. 211: *Daphnia magna* reproduction test, OECD guidelines for the testing of chemicals, section 2. OECD Publishing, Paris. https://doi.org/10.1787/9789264185203-en

OECD (2019) Guidance document on aquatic toxicity testing of difficult substances and mixtures, OECD series on testing and assessment. OECD Publishing, Paris. https://doi.org/10.1787/0ed2f88e-en

OECD (2025a) Test no. 203: fish, acute toxicity test, OECD guidelines for the testing of chemicals, section 2. OECD Publishing, Paris. https://doi.org/10.1787/9789264069961-en

OECD (2025b) Test no. 210: fish, early-life stage toxicity test, OECD guidelines for the testing of chemicals, section 2. OECD Publishing, Paris. https://doi.org/10.1787/9789264203785-en

Ogonowski M, Edlund U, Gorokhova E, Linde M, Ek K, Liewenborg B, Könnecke O, Navarro JRG, Breitholtz M (2018) Multi-level toxicity assessment of engineered cellulose nanofibrils in *Daphnia magna*. Nanotoxicology 12(6):509–521. https://doi.org/10.1080/17435390.2018.1464229

Ogura I, Matsuzawa T, Takata M (2020) Examples of detection and quantification of cellulose nanofibers. (in Japanese). https://riss.aist.go.jp/results-and-dissemin/776/

Ogura I, Sugiyama M, Tai R, Mano H, Matsuzawa T (2023) Optimization of microplate-based phenol-sulfuric acid method and application to the multi-sample measurements of cellulose nanofibers. Anal Biochem 681:11. https://doi.org/10.1016/j.ab.2023.115329

Ogura I, Moriyama A, Iizumi Y, Endoh S, Fujita K, Horie M, Okazaki T, Matsuzawa T (2025) Effect of gamma irradiation on cellulose nanofibers. J Wood Sci 71(1):37. https://doi.org/10.1186/s10086-025-02215-y

Ong KJ, Shatkin JA, Nelson K, Ede JD, Retsina T (2017) Establishing the safety of novel bio-based cellulose nanomaterials for commercialization. NanoImpact 6:19–29. https://doi.org/10.1016/j.impact.2017.03.002

Pengiran H, Kamaldin J, Fen LB, Yusob SAA (2022) Properties of kenaf cellulose nanofiber (CNF) as potential larvicide nanocarrier and its acute ecotoxicity against *Daphnia magna* and Dania rerio. J Nat Fibers 19(13):6756–6769. https://doi.org/10.1080/15440478.2021.1932673

Pereira MM, Mouton L, Yéprémian C, Couté A, Lo J, Marconcini JM, Ladeira LO, Raposo NRB, Brandão HM, Brayner R (2014) Ecotoxicological effects of carbon nanotubes and cellulose nanofibers in *Chlorella vulgaris*. J Nanobiotechnol 12(1):15. https://doi.org/10.1186/1477-3155-12-15

Rist S, Baun A, Hartmann NB (2017) Ingestion of micro- and nanoplastics in *Daphnia magna*—quantification of body burdens and assessment of feeding rates and reproduction. Environ Pollut 228:398–407. https://doi.org/10.1016/j.envpol.2017.05.048

Rusconi T, Riva L, Punta C, Solé M, Corsi I (2024) Environmental safety of nanocellulose: an acute *in vivo* study with marine mussels *Mytilus galloprovincialis*. Environ Sci Nano 11(1):61–77. https://doi.org/10.1039/D3EN00135K

Stoudmann N, Nowack B, Som C (2019) Prospective environmental risk assessment of nanocellulose for Europe. Environ Sci Nano 6(8):2520–2531. https://doi.org/10.1039/C9EN00472F

Tai R, Ogura I, Mano H (2022) Current status and considerations of ecotoxicity testing methods for cellulose nanofibers. Jpn J Environ Toxicol 25:32–47. (in Japanese)

Tai R, Ogura I, Okazaki T, Iizumi Y, Mano H (2024a) Acute toxicity tests of TEMPO-oxidized cellulose nanofiber using *Daphnia magna* and *Oryzias latipes*. Cellulose 31(4):2207–2220. https://doi.org/10.1007/s10570-024-05747-6

Tai R, Ogura I, Okazaki T, Iizumi Y, Mano H (2024b) Algal growth inhibition test with TEMPO-oxidized cellulose nanofibers. NanoImpact 34:100504. https://doi.org/10.1016/j.impact.2024.100504

US Environmental Protection Agency (US EPA) (2000) Methods for measuring the toxicity and bioaccumulation of sediment-associated contaminants with freshwater invertebrates, 2nd edn. United States Environmental Protection Agency Office of Water, EPA-600/R-99/064. https://archive.epa.gov/water/archive/polwaste/web/pdf/freshmanual.pdf. Accessed 28 Nov 2024

US Environmental Protection Agency (US EPA) (2002) Short-term methods for estimating the chronic toxicity of effluents and receiving waters to freshwater organisms, 4th edn. EPA-821-R-02-013. U.S. Environmental Protection Agency Office of Water, Washington DC. https://www.epa.gov/sites/production/files/2015-08/documents/short-term-chronic--freshwater-wet-manual_2002.pdf. Accessed 3 June 2021

Vartiainen J, Pöhler T, Sirola K, Pylkkänen L, Alenius H, Hokkinen J, Tapper U, Lahtinen P, Kapanen A, Putkisto K, Hiekkataipale P, Eronen P, Ruokolainen J, Laukkanen A (2011) Health and environmental safety aspects of friction grinding and spray drying of microfibrillated cellulose. Cellulose 18(3):775–786. https://doi.org/10.1007/s10570-011-9501-7

Wang Z, Song L, Ye N, Yu Q, Zhai Y, Zhang F, Vijver MG, Peijnenburg WJGM (2020) Oxidative stress actuated by cellulose nanocrystals and nanofibrils in aquatic organisms of different trophic levels. NanoImpact 17:10. https://doi.org/10.1016/j.impact.2020.100211

Wigger H, Kawecki D, Nowack B, Adam V (2020) Systematic consideration of parameter uncertainty and variability in probabilistic species sensitivity distributions. Integr Environ Assess Manag 16(2):211–222. https://doi.org/10.1002/ieam.4214

Chapter 9
Biodegradability: Effects of Nanosizing and Chemical Modification

Isamu Ogura

Abstract The increasing production and use of nanocellulose materials (NCMs) raise concerns regarding their environmental release and biodegradability. This chapter reviews existing literature on the biodegradability of cellulose nanofibrils (also referred to as cellulose nanofibers; CNFs) and cellulose nanocrystals (CNCs), and presents findings from the NEDO project, which specifically investigated the biodegradability of CNFs, with a focus on the effects of nanosizing and chemical modification. The results indicate that both CNFs and CNCs are generally biodegradable in a manner comparable to conventional cellulose. Although chemical modifications can influence biodegradability, general environmental tests conducted under the NEDO project demonstrate that TEMPO-oxidized, phosphorylated, and acetylated CNFs meet the criteria for ready biodegradability.

Keywords Nanocellulose · Cellulose nanofibrils · Nanomaterial safety · Ready biodegradability · Marine biodegradation · Environmental degradation · OECD guideline · Biodegradation tests · Environmental fate

9.1 Introduction

With the increasing practical application of nanocellulose materials (NCMs), their production volume and market distribution are also expected to increase. Consequently, the amounts of NCMs released into the environment may rise significantly through industrial and domestic wastewater pathways, as well as through outdoor applications such as construction, coatings, and agriculture. Although cellulose is a natural structural component of plants and is generally expected to biodegrade in the environment, nanosizing and chemical modification may influence its biodegradation behavior. This chapter reviews existing literature and presents

I. Ogura (✉)
Research Institute of Science for Safety and Sustainability (RISS), National Institute of Advanced Industrial Science and Technology (AIST), Tsukuba, Ibaraki, Japan
e-mail: i-ogura@aist.go.jp

I. Ogura, K. Fujita (eds.), *Nanocellulose Materials*,
https://doi.org/10.1007/978-981-92-2148-6_9

findings from the NEDO project (FY2017–2019) regarding the biodegradability of cellulose nanofibrils (also referred to as cellulose nanofibers; CNFs) and cellulose nanocrystals (CNCs).

9.2 Information from Existing Literature

Ong et al. (2017) conducted anaerobic biodegradation tests based on Organisation for Economic Co-operation and Development (OECD) test guideline (TG) 311 for lignin-coated CNFs (L-CNF) and lignin-coated CNCs (L-CNC). The anaerobic biodegradation rates were 51% for L-CNF and 35% for L-CNC, values comparable to or exceeding those reported for conventional cellulose. The authors also performed aerobic biodegradation tests following EPA OCSPP 835.3140. Under this protocol, a material is considered "readily biodegradable" if its biodegradation exceeds 60% within a 10-day window after reaching 10% degradation. L-CNF reached 10% degradation between Days 1 and 7, and achieved 71% by Day 14, thereby meeting the criterion for being readily biodegradable. L-CNC also reached 10% degradation between Days 1 and 7, attaining 41% by Day 14 and 68% by Day 21. While L-CNC was biodegradable, it did not fully satisfy the criteria for ready biodegradability.

Kümmerer et al. (2011) evaluated the biodegradability of CNCs (average cross-section 6 nm, length 180 nm) and starch nanoparticles alongside fullerenes and carbon nanotubes, using the OECD TG 301D closed bottle method. While fullerenes and carbon nanotubes showed no biodegradation, CNCs and starch nanoparticles exhibited biodegradability comparable to their macroscopic counterparts. Although neither material fully met the criterion for ready biodegradability (60% within 28 days), both degraded more rapidly than their bulk forms, likely due to their increased surface area.

O'Connor et al. (2014) conducted biodegradation tests on CNCs (nanocrystalline cellulose: NCC™) using OECD TG 301 and reported 42% biodegradation within the 10-day window.

Vikman et al. (2015) assessed the biodegradability and compostability of nanofibrillar cellulose (NFC)-based products—including NFC films, concentrated NFC, and paper products containing NFC—under controlled composting conditions. Compared with Whatman filter paper (cellulose), the relative biodegradation after 65 days reached 122% for NFC films, 93% for concentrated NFC, and 116% for NFC-containing paper products. All materials met the European standard EN 13432 requirement of ≥90% biodegradation relative to the reference material and were therefore considered biodegradable. Disintegration during composting was evaluated using a pilot-scale composting test modified from EN 14045, in which NFC films completely disintegrated within 3 weeks of composting, and NFC did not adversely affect the degradability of paper products containing NFC. Ecotoxicity during biodegradation of NFC products in a compost environment was evaluated using a bioluminescence test with the marine bacterium *Vibrio fischeri*, and no acute toxicity was observed for any of the tested samples.

9.3 Results of the NEDO Project

To gain insights into the biodegradability of CNFs under environmentally relevant conditions, biodegradation tests were conducted using the OECD TG 301C method (OECD 1992a) to determine whether CNFs can be classified as readily biodegradable (Kajihara et al. 2020). The OECD TG 301C test employs activated sludge cultured from samples collected at ten locations across Japan, including surface waters from rivers, lakes, and coastal areas, as well as return sludge from sewage treatment plants. This approach is designed to assess biodegradation by microorganisms commonly present in diverse environmental media.

Under OECD TG 301C, a substance is considered "readily biodegradable" if its biodegradation, quantified as biochemical oxygen demand (BOD), reaches 60% or more within a 28-day test period. The results of the biodegradation tests for CNFs and reference cellulose materials are summarized in Table 9.1.

TEMPO-oxidized CNFs, phosphorylated CNFs, mechanically fibrillated CNFs, and acetylated CNFs all exhibited biodegradation exceeding 60% and were therefore classified as readily biodegradable. Although the degree of biodegradation of cellulose powder (Avicel PH-101) varied depending on the test conditions, it was nevertheless classified as readily biodegradable. In cases where biodegradation did not exceed 60% within the 28-day test period, the samples were nevertheless observed to be undergoing active biodegradation.

The degradation degree of acetylated pulp was below 60%; however, this result was attributable to one of three replicate samples ($n = 3$) exhibiting negligible biodegradation (2%), while the remaining two samples showed substantial

Table 9.1 Results of biodegradability tests using the OECD TG 301C method (Kajihara et al. 2020)

Test material	Test 1	Test 2	Test 3
TEMPO-oxidized CNFs	Readily biodegradable	–	–
Phosphorylated CNFs	–	Readily biodegradable	–
Mechanically fibrillated CNFs	–	Readily biodegradable	–
Acetylated pulp (DS: 0.69)	–	–	Readily biodegradable
Acetylated lignin-containing (ligno-)CNFs (DS: 0.69)	–	–	Readily biodegradable
Cellulose powder (Avicel PH-101)	Readily biodegradable	Readily biodegradable	Readily biodegradable
Cellulose acetate (DS: 2.4)	–	–	Not readily biodegradable

"–" indicates that the test was not conducted

DS degree of substitution

Tests 1–3 were conducted during different periods, and the activated sludge used in each test was sourced independently biodegradation (80% and 77%). Based on this distribution of results, acetylated pulp was judged to be readily biodegradable. In contrast, cellulose acetate (degree of substitution, DS = 2.4), used as a reference material, did not exhibit biodegradation and was therefore classified as not readily biodegradable.

In addition, biodegradability in seawater was evaluated using a modified version of OECD TG 306 (OECD 1992b), in which biodegradation was assessed by BOD instead of dissolved organic carbon (DOC). Due to the variability in microbial composition in seawater, this test is prone to fluctuations and potential false-negative results. Furthermore, factors such as nutrient supplementation and high test-substance concentrations may limit the ability of the test to accurately simulate marine environmental conditions. Consequently, a positive result indicates potential biodegradability in seawater, whereas a negative result does not necessarily imply that the test substance is nonbiodegradable under marine conditions.

Using this modified marine biodegradation test, TEMPO-oxidized CNFs, mechanically fibrillated CNFs, unmodified lignin-containing (ligno-)CNFs, acetylated ligno-CNFs (DS = 0.40), and acetylated ligno-CNFs (DS = 0.84) all exhibited biodegradation exceeding 60%, indicating their potential biodegradability in marine environments.

9.4 Summary

Based on existing literature and findings from the NEDO project, both CNFs and CNCs are generally considered biodegradable in a manner comparable to conventional cellulose. Although chemical modifications may affect their biodegradability, results from general environmental biodegradation tests conducted under the NEDO project demonstrated that TEMPO-oxidized, phosphorylated, and acetylated CNFs meet the criteria for ready biodegradability.

References

Kajihara H, Gamo M, Oguri T (2020) Chapter 6: degradation after environmental release, examples of emission and exposure assessment of cellulose nanofibers and their applied products (in Japanese). https://riss.aist.go.jp/results-and-dissemin/776/

Kümmerer K, Menz J, Schubert T, Thielemans W (2011) Biodegradability of organic nanoparticles in the aqueous environment. Chemosphere 82(10):1387–1392. https://doi.org/10.1016/j.chemosphere.2010.11.069

O'Connor B, Berry R, Goguen R (2014) Chapter 10: risks, regulation, and management micro and Nano Technologies. In: Commercialization of cellulose nanocrystal (NCC™) production: a business case focusing on the importance of proactive EHS management, Nanotechnology environmental health and safety, 2nd edn. William Andrew, pp 225–246

OECD (1992a) Test no. 301: ready biodegradability, OECD guidelines for the testing of chemicals, section 3. OECD Publishing, Paris. https://doi.org/10.1787/9789264070349-en

OECD (1992b) Test no. 306: biodegradability in seawater, OECD guidelines for the testing of chemicals, section 3. OECD Publishing, Paris. https://doi.org/10.1787/9789264070486-en
Ong KJ, Shatkin JA, Nelson K, Ede JD, Retsina T (2017) Establishing the safety of novel bio-based cellulose nanomaterials for commercialization. NanoImpact 6:19–29. https://doi.org/10.1016/j.impact.2017.03.002
Vikman M, Vartiainen J, Tsitko I, Korhonen P (2015) Biodegradability and compostability of nanofibrillar cellulose-based products. J Polym Environ 23(2):206–215. https://doi.org/10.1007/s10924-014-0694-3

Correction to: Nanocellulose Materials

Isamu Ogura and Katsuhide Fujita

Correction to: I. Ogura, K. Fujita (eds.), *Nanocellulose Materials*, https://doi.org/10.1007/978-981-92-2148-6

The original version of the book was inadvertently published with incorrect copyright holder name. The copyright holder name has been corrected as The Editor(s) (if applicable) and The Author(s).

The updated versions of this book can be found at
https://doi.org/10.1007/978-981-92-2148-6

I. Ogura, K. Fujita (eds.), *Nanocellulose Materials*,
https://doi.org/10.1007/978-981-92-2148-6_10

Index

A
Aerodynamic particle sizer (APS), 101, 106, 107
Algal growth inhibition tests, 138, 140–142, 147
Ames test, 3, 11, 13, 14, 16, 18
Aqueous counter collision (ACC), 62, 137, 141, 143, 144, 147

B
Battery tests, 15

C
Carbon nanotubes (CNTs), 3, 4, 10, 27–30, 42, 56, 66, 67, 96, 103, 114, 152
Cellulose microfibrils (CMFs), 12, 14, 15, 48, 49
Cellulose nanocrystals (CNCs), 1–3, 6, 10, 12–16, 40, 42–50, 59, 60, 64, 66, 67, 74, 76, 82–87, 89, 94, 97–102, 106, 112, 113, 125–129, 152, 154
Cellulose nanofibrils/cellulose nanofibers (CNFs), 1, 2, 10, 13, 16, 24, 40, 74, 82, 94, 122, 152
Chemokines, 3, 30, 32–34, 44, 45, 47, 49
Chromosomal aberration test, 3, 11–14, 17–19
Comet assays, 12–16
Comprehensive gene expression analysis, 32, 48
Condensation particle counter (CPC), 98–101, 104–107
Cultured cell test, 34
Cytokines, 3, 13, 16, 32–34, 44–49, 57, 58, 60, 63, 64, 75, 76, 86

D
Daphnia magna reproduction test, 129, 130, 136, 141, 143, 147
Daphnia sp. acute immobilisation test, 143
Dynamic probabilistic material flow analysis (DPMFA), 132–134

E
EC_{50}, 124–128, 141, 143

F
Fish, acute toxicity test, 136, 143
Fish, early-life stage toxicity test, 136, 143, 147

G
Genotoxicity, 2–4, 10–20, 42, 44, 48, 49, 88

I
Inhalation toxicity test, 40
International Organization for Standardization (ISO), 7, 55, 95, 100, 123
Intratracheal instillation tests, 50
In vitro test, 16
In vivo tests, 133

I. Ogura, K. Fujita (eds.), *Nanocellulose Materials*,
https://doi.org/10.1007/978-981-92-2148-6

L

LC_{50}, 124–128, 141, 143
LD_{50}, 82, 85–87, 89
Lipopolysaccharide (LPS), 16, 57

M

Macrophages, 4, 13–16, 26, 27, 32–34, 41–45, 47, 49, 58–60, 62–65, 67, 88
Mesothelial cells, 24–26, 28, 30, 32–34
Mesothelioma, 2, 3, 10, 24–34, 97
Microcrystalline cellulose (MCC), 13, 16, 17, 40–42, 82, 87, 123, 124
Microfibrillated cellulose/microfibrillar cellulose (MFC), 2, 75, 76, 98–100, 123, 124, 131
Micronucleus, 3, 11–17, 19, 49
Micronucleus test in erythrocytes, 3, 17, 19
Mouse lymphoma TK assay, 18
Multi-walled carbon nanotubes (MWCNTs), 10, 17, 24, 27–30, 33, 42–44, 46, 49, 54–57, 60, 66, 67, 97

N

Nanocellulose/nanocellulose materials (NCMs), 1–5, 7, 10, 11, 15, 17–19, 24, 40–42, 46–67, 74, 75, 77, 78, 87, 94, 97–98, 101, 112, 113, 115–117, 122–128, 130–135, 148, 151
Nanocrystalline cellulose (NCC), 100, 101, 123, 124, 152
Nanofibrillated cellulose/nanofibrillar cellulose (NFC/NCF), 2, 14, 43, 44, 48, 49, 74, 152
National Institute for Occupational Safety and Health (NIOSH), 95–98, 101
National Institute of Advanced Industrial Science and Technology (AIST), 2, 50, 66
New Energy and Industrial Technology Development Organization (NEDO), 2–4, 6, 17–20, 24, 30–33, 40, 41, 43, 47, 50–67, 74–78, 82, 88, 89, 94, 97, 103–117, 122, 135–148, 152–154
No-observed-adverse-effect level (NOAEL), 60, 82–85, 87, 89, 125, 128, 130
No observed effect concentration (NOEC), 125, 128, 131, 141, 143–145

O

OECD TGs, 3, 4, 11–14, 16, 18–19, 50, 60, 76–78, 82–88, 123, 129–131, 136, 140, 152–154
Optical particle counter (OPC), 99–102, 104–107
Organisation for Economic Co-operation and Development (OECD), 3, 7, 11, 18, 19, 40, 60, 75, 77, 82, 122, 130, 135, 136, 140, 152–154
Oropharyngeal aspiration, 40, 42–46
Oxidative stress, 15, 25, 26, 32, 33, 41, 42, 46–49, 64, 126, 127, 129

P

Predicted environmental concentration (PEC), 132–135
Predicted no-effect concentrations (PNECs), 6, 122, 136, 144, 147
Probabilistic species sensitivity distribution (PSSD), 132–134

R

Reactive oxygen species (ROS), 15, 26, 48–50, 62, 76, 128
Respirable dust, 55, 95–98, 104–106, 109, 112, 113
Risk characterization ratio (RCR), 132–134

S

Scanning electron microscope (SEM), 99, 100, 103–107, 109, 112
Scanning mobility particle sizer (SMPS), 98–102, 106, 107

T

TEMPO, 125
Test guideline (TG), 11–14, 40, 75, 82, 86, 129, 152
Transmission electron microscope (TEM), 49, 50, 59, 64, 107

U

Uncertainty factor (UF), 144, 145, 147
United States Environmental Protection Agency (USEPA), 139

MIX
Papier aus verantwortungsvollen Quellen
Paper from responsible sources
FSC® C105338

If you have any concerns about our products,
you can contact us on
ProductSafety@springernature.com

In case Publisher is established outside the EU,
the EU authorized representative is:
Springer Nature Customer Service Center GmbH
Europaplatz 3, 69115 Heidelberg, Germany

Printed by Libri Plureos GmbH
in Hamburg, Germany